MEDITATIONS FOR
LIVING IN BALANCE

MEDITATIONS FOR LIVING IN BALANCE

DAILY SOLUTIONS
FOR PEOPLE WHO DO TOO MUCH

ANNE WILSON SCHAEF, PH.D.

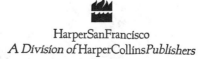

HarperSanFrancisco
A Division of HarperCollins*Publishers*

HarperCollins Web site: http://www.harpercollins.com

HarperCollins®, 📖®, and HarperSanFrancisco™ are trademarks of HarperCollins Publishers, Inc.

FIRST EDITION

Library of Congress Cataloging-in-Publication Data
Schaef, Anne Wilson.
Meditations for living in balance: daily solutions for people
  who do too much/by Anne Wilson Schaef.—1st ed.
    p. cm.
  ISBN 0—06—251643—4 (pbk.)
  Spiritual life—Meditations. 2. Conduct of life—
  Meditations. 3. Devotional calendars. I. Title.
  BL624.2 S29 2001
  158.1'28—dc21   00—039619
        07 BANTA 10 9 8 7

To all who seek
spiritual and functional balance in their lives.

INTRODUCTION

I bring this book to you as one who is walking with you on the journey to find meaning and fulfillment in this busy, sometimes chaotic life that each of us has chosen.

Regardless of who we are or what we do, we live in a fast-paced, technological world of growing globalization where doing too much is the norm and moments of quiet peace and calm are more precious than any commodity that can be found on the Internet.

In spite of this, we are human beings who are spiritual, emotional, and feeling creatures who need much more than chaotic rushing and materialism. We have needs, many needs. We need to grow. We need to be as fully alive as we can be. We need to know and respond to the depths of our spiritual selves and resonate with that which is beyond ourselves. We need to be productive. We need to be loving. We need to be connected. We need to participate in our lives in a way that is full and meaningful.

All too often when we think of living in balance, we approach balance in the same frantic, rushing way that we approach the rest of our lives. We want to balance work and home. We want to balance relationships. We want to work out and exercise and eat good food. We want to stay healthy so that we can do more. We want to fill everything up, our selves, our time, our activities, our relationships, and our lives. If we are not careful, we will add balancing our lives to our already long list of doing too much.

Before I go any further, I want to say something about the concept of balance itself. One of the main difficulties we create for ourselves in trying to live our lives is our dualistic thinking. We think in terms of this or that. We set up our lives in abstract dualisms. We want to balance work and family and delude ourselves into thinking that when we do that, life will be fine. We forget about alone time, friendships, entertainment, spiritual growth, exercise, and fun. When we think in dualisms, we see ourselves and our lives as two-dimensional and we limit and destroy our possibilities. Dualisms do two things: (1) they distort a very complex set of circumstances into a simplistic set of pairs, thereby lulling us into a false sense of security, and (2) they feed our illusion of control. Neither of these adds to our growth, learning, serenity, or happiness.

This book will not take that simplistic solution. I believe that we, as spiritual beings, are capable of so much more.

In this book, balance will not be imaged as the weights held by justice or as a seesaw. Instead, balance will be pushed further toward a multivariate, multidimensional state of being more akin to harmony.

I share these paragraphs taken from the Desana people of the Amazon. They tell one of their creation stories.

> Through this act of creation, the Sun gave shape to the world *with the power of his yellow light and gave it life and stability.* This *stability* in nature, the Desana are eager to emphasize, is not merely a static seesaw state of balance. Rather, it is a dynamic state embodying a vast and continuous multiplicity of exchanges among all the components of

the Sun's wondrous creation—not unlike what a contemporary ecologist might refer to as a "biological equilibrium."

According to Desana, this inherent *stability* of the natural world is rooted in a vast web of reciprocal relationships that have always existed between all elements in nature. A reciprocity between the earth—with its myriad mountains and forests and rivers—and the first forms of life—the animals, the plants, the Desana people—exists in harmony with all the rest of the universe. For as traditional Desana tell it, the *Sun planned his creation very well, and it was perfect.*[1]

The issue for me here and what I am trying to communicate is a concept of balance as harmony—living in balance as being and living in harmony with your universe, wherever and however you find yourself.

Balance (harmony) is never static. One does not achieve a state of balance that, once achieved, will stay that way forever. We may want to get our bodies in shape—and we can. Yet those bodies are a process, and being in shape is ongoing, not something one accomplishes and then moves on to bigger and better things. We may want to get our cars or our houses just the way we want them, and we can do that. And the balance we seek for our houses or cars is fleeting at best. Life is just like our checkbooks. We need to learn the tools for bringing them back into balance, for once we get them balanced, they will only have a possibility of staying that way if

1. David Suzuki and Peter Knudtson, *Wisdom of the Elders*, (New York: Bantam Books, 1992). From the authors of that book: "Italicized words in the story of the Desana denote direct quotations from Native sources or scholarly interpretations of them. In the original sources, Native words are encoded in a variety of specialized linguistic systems; here, for the sake of uniformity and readability, they have been simplified to their approximate English equivalents."

we never use them again. Living in harmony is an ongoing process.

This book, then, is about balance as harmony. To achieve this living harmony, we need to let go of some of the old ideas, beliefs, and practices that have brought imbalance and disharmony in our lives. We need to let go of the dysfunctional simplification of dualistic thinking. We need to open ourselves and stretch ourselves to the harmonious balance that dwells within and around each of us if we can find it. We cannot keep harmonious balance. We can only learn to return to it as quickly and easily as possible.

This book opens the doors to possibilities of harmonious balance.

Each entry starts with challenging and important words of wisdom. This is followed by words related to the quote that open doors for our movement toward harmonious balance. These words are then followed by an action that will offer the possibility of movement toward greater balance. Although I have ended almost every day with actions we can take to balance our lives, these actions are not suggestions that will add to our overdoing; they are simply steps we can take to come to solutions with our doing-too-much imbalance. All of the pieces are important. Just as each day is a movement toward balance, the whole book is a movement toward harmonious, balanced living.

These pages not only offer food for our too-busy, high-pressured beings, spirits, and lives, they also offer tools and practical ways of living more sanely and fully within our busy lives. We need food for our minds and beings every day, and we also need practical tools and practices that will help us to walk through the doors we have creaked open and move forward to more creative, fulfilling, and harmonious lives. Remember, as I always say: "The practical should always be in the service of the important."

I hope you enjoy using this book as much as I enjoyed writing it. As is usual in the process of writing, I learned much and was pushed to move through false dualisms and static notions that supported disharmony and imbalance.

When we do too much, let it be in the service of returning us to harmonious balance.

MEDITATIONS FOR
LIVING IN BALANCE

A CHANGING BALANCE

Sameness is not always balancing.

ANONYMOUS

Some of us have bought into the illusion that we can work hard to get our lives organized and "balanced" and they will stay that way forever. Not so!

Sameness is not balance. One of the givens of being human beings (like it or not!) is that we are constantly granted the opportunity and *mandate* to grow, to learn, and to change. Our houses and our cars keep trying to teach us that all material objects are in a constant state of disintegration, and we don't want to believe them. How much more difficult is it to see ourselves and our world this way!

Balance will never be attained once and for all. That's just the way life is. That is the human condition. We can either accept it or keep trying to live in illusion. Some of us may choose the third option of doing both—accepting it for a while or for some things and then not for others. We do make it rough on ourselves, don't we?

The most balancing thing we can do for ourselves is accept the joy of feeling balanced when we do, recognizing that the balancing and rebalancing of ourselves is an ongoing process that offers us a minute-by-minute opportunity.

Take a look at any aspect of your life you believe you have "balanced" or are trying to keep the same and see if this is causing you stress. If so, try putting on new glasses and celebrating the balance that is there while accepting the change that is just around the corner.

HAPPINESS

Happiness makes up in height for what it lacks in length.
ROBERT FROST

We too often focus our attention on what happiness *isn't* rather than on what it *is*. Our biggest complaint is that it never lasts. We never have this complaint about sadness, yet both are feelings that will come and go. Happiness just gets its job done faster. That's all.

Let's take a look at happiness.

Happiness is that brief sigh of a moment that delivers a glow of peace and serenity. Happiness is that tiny point of a feeling in our chest that radiates itself a million times throughout our being. Happiness is that "pause" that refreshes our spirit, allowing us to plunge back into the rigors of our lives with renewed vigor. Happiness is that precise moment that allows us to experience—even if briefly—that we are a part of a vastness our minds will never comprehend.

Don't knock the brevity of happiness. Rejoice in its existence.

Most of us have many brief moments of happiness every day—regardless of what else is going on. Practice noticing them.

THE IMPORTANT

I've learned that the great challenge of life is to decide what's important and to disregard everything else.

ANONYMOUS

We are such amazing creatures, we human beings. We get so busy and so involved with the rush of living that all too often we spend our most productive years in the pursuit of things that are not really important to us. When one stands back and gets some perspective on this situation, it seems quite foolish indeed. Yet, when we are in the middle of it, whatever "unimportant" activity we are investing our time and energy into seems quite legitimate. For some of us, it is only as we start to grow older that we realize that the important has been put aside for the expedient. No wonder our lives feel out of balance to us sometimes. We are not investing in our "importants" and we are squandering our valuable days, weeks, and years on things that really don't matter that much to us.

Luckily, we always have the option to stop, to back off, and to reevaluate what is important for us.

Devote one day a year to taking stock. See how you are spending your time. List what is important to you and see how the two relate. Always be open to seeing the excuses you are using to justify doing "unimportant" things. Share this information with someone close to you.

DISCOMFORT

The simplest kind of guidance [critique] comes every day, and many times a day in the form of discomfort.

BARBARA ANN BRENNAN

Most of us would like to believe that we have some kind of guidance even if we struggle with the concept of God. Not only would we like to have this guidance to fall back on when self-will proves inadequate, we would like it to be in a loud, clear voice or in unmistakable visions. Too bad! Often it comes in the form of a slight discomfort.

I know a woodworker who waited until the last minute to make all his Christmas presents. He was getting very close to Christmas when he began to have trouble with a certain piece of wood. It just wouldn't work right. He had misgivings about the wood, his tools, the lathe—everything. Yet he persevered, working on one piece for several days. The day before Christmas Eve the whole piece fell apart. His mistake? He hadn't listened to his discomfort. He pushed on through his uneasiness when he could have started a new project. He ignored his guidance and it was costly.

Feelings of discomfort are some of our wisest sources of information.

Practice noticing and heeding your discomfort.

PROVERBS

The laden almond tree by the wayside is sure to be bitter.
JAPANESE PROVERB

I just love proverbs! A really good proverb communicates a depth of wisdom that tickles our right brain and intuition while sometimes leaving our left, logical brain at a bit of a loss to articulate what the proverb means. Deep inside, we *know* what it means as it strikes and causes some profound inner wisdom to resonate within us. Yet, the true meaning goes far beyond what our logical, rational mind can provide. A good proverb guides our *being*, not just our *thinking*, and in so doing opens up ancient paths of wisdom for the living of our lives.

Take the above Japanese proverb, for example. Of course, we all get it that if an easily accessible tree is heavily laden and not picked, the fruit (or nuts) must not be any good. It also warns us not to be fooled by appearances while at the same time trusting appearances and the obvious. On yet another level, it encourages us to look beyond the easily accessible and not to be satisfied until we have what may be better fruit even if we have to work for it. And on another level . . .

Put more proverbs in your life and share them with the children you know.

WASTE

Waste is a spiritual thing and harms the soul as well as the pocket book.

KATHLEEN NORRIS

When we are thinking of what balances and what unbalances our lives, it's important to take a look at waste. When we look at waste as "a spiritual thing that harms the soul," it takes on a very personal meaning. It is no longer an abstract concept that "someone" should do something about. Viewed from this perspective, waste enters into the very fiber of our being and demands attention. The spiritual aspect of waste requires that we stop to see how our wasting contributes to our feelings of being unbalanced.

For example, did you ever notice how good you feel when you creatively use leftovers rather than throwing them out? Most of us get a certain glow of positive self-satisfaction when we put even the tiniest effort into recycling.

Although we may feel like we can afford it, wasting time, wasting money, wasting ourselves, and wasting things just doesn't feel good.

Zero in on one or two ways you are "wasting" that bug you and make some changes.

LONELINESS AND SOLITUDE

Loneliness is the poverty of self; solitude is the richness of self.
MAY SARTON

Loneliness is different from time alone. It is different from solitude. Feelings of loneliness are often the marvelous signals that our inner beings send us that we have left ourselves. No one can *make* us lonely. We may be in situations where it is extremely difficult to stay with ourselves. And, loneliness is most often a loneliness for ourselves.

Regardless of the external circumstances, when we are in touch with ourselves and living in our bodies, loneliness is next to impossible.

We may miss someone; that's okay. Missing someone means we have let that person become an important part of our lives, and that's a good thing to do. Our missing them is the inward awareness that we have let ourselves love and be loved.

Missing *ourselves* is another matter entirely. When we miss ourselves, we have lost a most important and intimate connection. It is only through ourselves that we can connect with a power greater than ourselves.

When we are connected with ourselves and our spiritual being, we need and welcome solitude.

When you stop to realize that you feel lonely, take a look at ways you have given yourself away. An apology to yourself might be in order.

KNOWING GOD

God is like a mirror. The mirror never changes but everybody who looks at it sees something different.

RABBI HAROLD KUSHNER

We intuitively know that having a connection to God helps us find inner harmony. Yet, there is so much hostility and consternation in the world that revolves around whose perception of God is right. How exhausting!

Do we really believe that God (or whatever one wants to call it) is so simple that one person or group of people can get the whole picture? It has taken years and years and hundreds of people to get the meager knowledge that we have about the atom. How much more complex is God?

Alcoholics Anonymous refers to "the God of our understanding." What a peaceful way to approach knowing God. If each of us looks into a mirror and sees a piece of God, then we need all the pieces we can get—and then some. Whoever we are, whatever we are, we have the understanding we need within us. It's that simple.

If we need to know and understand more about God, we can *listen* to others as well as to all creation. We are surrounded by spiritual scholars, educated and uneducated.

Some day, when rushing is not an issue, stop to see what you know about God within yourself. Not what you have been taught, not what you think you should know, not what others know. You have your own information. Trust it.

LIFELONG LEARNING

I'm still learning.

MICHELANGELO

Life cannot be compressed into little blocks that are separate and distinct from one another. Nor can learning be broken up into convenient blocks discretely separate. Life and learning are both processes. We never "get there" in either one.

We have been led to believe that we can get educated and then we *are* educated. Not true! There is no way we can ever know ahead of time all the skills we will need for a lifetime. Also, there is no way another person or system can know what each person needs to walk the path she or he must walk. We can gain certain basic skills, and true balance in learning comes from its continuous process.

Continuous learning is one of the ways we stay young. Continuous learning adds balance to the knowledge and skills we have already mastered. Continuous learning opens new doors for humility. Nothing is a better ego restrainer than being "new" at something, anything. Being a beginner does not massage our ego; it cleans it. And *everyone's* ego needs cleaning once in a while.

Start learning something new today. Preferably something you may not be good at.

HONOR AND MORALITY

Laws can never do what morality [honor] is intended to do.
ANNE WILSON SCHAEF

What illusions we have spun to convince ourselves that we are safe and in control! What complex devices we have concocted to feed our desire for stasis and security! What complexities we have engendered to drug ourselves into complacency! How important it is to take the time to determine what our personal morality is and to live by it!

It takes time to clearly define our personal morality . . . to learn to be clear about what is honorable for us. For example, most of us are taught as children that we should not lie. Yet we see dishonesty all around us. All too often, our role models say one thing and do another. Hopefully, at some point in our lives, we have to move from "out there" to "in here." We need to redefine ourselves with what is honorable for *us*. Perhaps others can cross a line that would not be right for us. That's *their* problem.

At some point, we can no longer delude ourselves into thinking that if it is legal it is all right even if we know it is wrong for us. Personal balance is a personal matter. Only we can bring ourselves into personal balance, and this balance is dependent upon what is honorable for us.

Take a look at the things you try to get away with and see if they are honorable for you. Do they add to your sense of wholeness? Do they deplete your sense of wholeness?

EXPERIMENTING WITH LIFE

Our own life is the instrument with which we experiment with truth.

THICH NHAT HANH

To "experiment with truth" means that we make mistakes. If we completely knew truth, we would not have to experiment with it . . . we would "be there." Yet, this human life is not so constructed as to "be there." That's why it is a *process* and not a *thing.*

Our lives are set up so that we are given an ongoing process in which to participate. That participation is the way we experiment with the ultimate truth, which can only be glimpsed from moment to moment. Yet, it is only known in seemingly disconnected fragments and pieces that come together in a recognizable picture when we least expect it.

Our task is to learn to seek balance as we participate in the process of experimenting with truth. All too often, we fall into the illusion that if we just stop, quit participating, and take control, we will be all right. Nothing could be further from the truth! Not participating in our lives and trying to control them is a tempting solution and one that never produces what we want.

Life is something like a balance board consisting of those half balls glued to a board. The idea is to practice balance, not to be static.

Take a look at something you have been trying to control and let yourself see what a ridiculous solution trying to control it is. Then, if you can, try letting go and see what happens.

FORGIVENESS

People are more than the worst thing they have ever done in their lives.

HELEN PREJEAN

One of the most debilitating concepts that emerged in the late twentieth century is that people are static . . . a modified static, I might add. There is a tendency to believe that people who have done something wrong or bad are bad people and will always be bad people. There is a deep, usually hidden and unspoken, belief that people can't really change and that they are no more than "the worst thing they have ever done in their lives." This belief results in a great deal of secret-keeping and the need to try to keep our pasts hidden. The modified static comes in with people who are perceived as "good." They always have the possibility of turning "bad" in the cultural wisdom.

Let's look at building a new cultural wisdom. What if people are a process designed to learn and grow from their mistakes? What if the "worst" things we have done can be the greatest opportunities for learning and growing? What if we really can grow and change, and the worst that we have done is the most important because it offers the opportunity for ourselves and others to learn and practice the process of forgiveness? The process of forgiveness is one of the most important balancing processes we can learn in this life, and self-forgiveness is perhaps the most difficult of all.

Are there things you have done for which you need to forgive yourself so you can move on? Inventory some of them.

GOD-TALK

Why is it when we talk to God, we're said to be praying—but when God talks to us, we're schizophrenic?

LILY TOMLIN

Good humor is when we have an opportunity to laugh at the greatest truths so they have an opportunity to sneak past our rational, logical brains and seep into our beings, where it counts.

"Science" has set up a system in which we feel uncomfortable with anything that cannot be observed, counted, and measured. God talking with us seemingly falls into that category, so this experience has ceased to be a part of polite conversations except in some institutions.

Yet, to those willing to listen, God talks to us all the time. One of God's voices is a "knowing" inside. We don't know *why* we know or *how* we know. We just know. (Trusting our knowings is where the hard part comes in.) God speaks to us through our feelings. Feelings are very important vehicles of God communication. When we are out of touch with our feelings, we are probably out of touch with God.

God speaks to us through other people, books, songs, and the wind. Chatter interferes with our ability to hear God-talk.

Do you trust God-talk? Do you have an attitude of interested listening for God-talk? Practice being ready.

LYING

Never lie to a child.

ANNE WILSON SCHAEF

Who knows what damage is done when we lie to a child?

There is, of course, the abuse of trust and the distortion of reality for the child. Yet, what happens to *us* when we lie to a child?

Lying is one of the seemingly simple acts we do to ourselves that have many resounding implications.

When we lie to a child, we have taken the trust of someone smaller and maybe even more vulnerable than ourselves and violated that trust. We have become a bully. We are a bully who is willing to abuse our role as adult and protector and exploit the trust that has been given to us. We cannot participate in that kind of exploitation without losing faith in ourselves.

When we lie, we send a message to ourselves that we are someone who cannot be trusted and so we cease to trust ourselves. With the simple act of lying to a child, we have set up a chain reaction in ourselves that is both painful and destructive.

We may try to convince ourselves that our lying is protecting the child and usually we are protecting the coward in ourselves. We rob the child of learning to cope with life and we rob ourselves of being an honorable person. In the long run, it's never worth it.

Be very careful what you say to a child. Your honor is at stake.

PROCRASTINATION

You never find yourself until you face the truth.

PEARL BAILEY

Maybe tomorrow. Maybe *they* weren't ready to hear the truth. Maybe the truth is too stark or too difficult. Maybe it will confirm their belief (secretly held by us) that we are nasty people if we tell the truth. Maybe the truth isn't necessary. Maybe the truth will only make things worse, so it is better to say nothing. Maybe—maybe—maybe . . .

The truth is that we can procrastinate about anything—even about telling the truth. Procrastination is one of the great imbalancers of life. We become so paralyzed by analyzing what might be possible or not possible, what the consequences may or may not be, what we can do or not do, that we move into a kind of paralysis that completely immobilizes us.

We look for salvation in the proper time, the proper timing, the proper way, or the proper setting, thereby avoiding any action that might alter our paralysis.

Although we may become accustomed to procrastination, we never become easy with it. Its very nature is to nag, tease, disturb, and haunt. Procrastination is not our friend.

Go straighten up your underwear drawer.

COMMUNICATION

May every disciple take care not to cling to words, as if they were a perfect expression of the meaning; because truth is not in the letters. When a man points to something with the finger, the tip of the finger may be mistaken for the thing pointed at. In the same way the ignorant and simple-minded are like children, incapable of giving up the idea that in the finger-tip of words the actual meaning is contained.

LAMA ANAGARIKA GOVINDA

We have made great progress on our journey to balance when we realize that words are always inaccurate expressions of the meaning we hope to communicate. No one is more aware of this than writers. We take seriously the responsibility to communicate as accurately as possible while realizing that our readers may be fixated on the tip of the finger. How much more can be transcended if we are not only aware of the tip of the finger, the space and the silence between the finger and the object, and the wondrousness of the object itself. Humility follows any attempt to communicate clearly, accurately, and meaningfully.

Our best hope is to take responsibility for what we say and to speak from the heart. Heartspeak is easier to understand for those who truly want to hear.

When we understand that there is more to communication than meets the eye, we can be gentler with ourselves.

Wait until you are ready to speak. Then try speaking clearly from the heart, not just the head.

HELLOS

I don't like the word stranger. *It doesn't fit for me anymore. The more centered I am in myself and the more "connected" I feel, it just doesn't fit.*

CONNIE

The word *stranger* conjures up some foreign and frightening images. When we see people as strangers, we assume that they are different from us and that we have nothing in common with them.

The truth is that most of us are more similar to each other than we are different. As human beings, we have great, wonderful differences that are rich and exciting *and* we are also very similar.

When we start noticing and really seeing people, we begin to become aware of our similarities.

Did you ever notice that when you begin to smile and nod at people, many of them smile back? A simple hello goes a long way toward establishing feelings of connectedness between oneself and others. Probably the most exciting and important aspect of starting to say random hellos is that we begin to change inside. We begin to feel happier. We begin to like ourselves better. And, we just may start sensing more positive energy coming our way.

Loneliness is a decision and a state of mind. We have a choice.

Start saying random hellos and see what happens.

LIFE'S TEACHERS

To learn from every man and to accept the truth from all who speak it.
FROM THE LAWS AND CUSTOMS OF ISRAEL

The world is full of teachers and sometimes sadly lacking in learners.

One of the ways we limit ourselves is by believing that only certain kinds of people can be our teachers or have anything that we need. Our range of teachers is directly proportional to the openness of our minds. In fact, some of our most important teachers are those to whom we have come to feel superior.

When we are open, our teachers appear in the most amazing places.

I am a person who dribbles. No matter how much I try not to, I dribble on my front. I used to believe that I would either have to wear spotted clothes or throw them out. Over the years, two people came into my life who saved my wardrobe and my clothing budget.

The first was a baby-sitter who had worked for a dry cleaners. She told me that one of the most effective tools for removing spots is your fingernail. It's true! Just work at it. Later, a student of mine told me of a little green German soap that removes almost all stains in anything. Again, right on. Between the two, I am usually spotless (except right after meals, of course).

Some may say these examples are not wisdom. Please remember that wisdom comes in all shapes and forms. Look carefully!

Today, try stretching your open-mindedness and look for teachers in places that were heretofore viewed as strange or impossible for learning.

SPIRITUALITY

Our deep spirituality is the best balancer.
                                            ANNE WILSON SCHAEF

When we are busy, we rarely think of spirituality. We reserve spirituality for a designated hour on weekends, for other quiet, saintly times of meditation, or for walks in nature. We often have made every attempt possible to keep spirituality compartmentalized and separate from our "real" life.

Unfortunately, spirituality just doesn't work that way. Spirituality is not something we choose or don't choose. Spirituality is who we are. Spirituality is the ground of our being that makes operating possible. It is not just the core out of which we operate; it is the basic process that makes functioning at all possible. How foolish we are when we think we are too busy for spirituality! Our spirituality is what makes it possible for us to be busy.

Spirituality is participation.

When we participate in our lives we are being spiritual. It's as simple as that. We can't run away from our spirituality—it goes with us everywhere.

SUPPORT

For every one of us that succeeds, it's because there's somebody there to show you the way out. The light doesn't necessarily have to be in your family; for me it was teachers and school.

OPRAH WINFREY

We have such an illusion of the self-made person in this society. Whatever it is we do or whoever we become, all of us have had help along the way. Help may not always have looked the way we expected or wanted it to look. All too often we think of help as warm, nurturing support. And while that kind of help is wonderful, all the warm, nurturing support in the world cannot teach us the same lessons as those we learn coming up against a worthy adversary or someone who does not like us much.

Years later, we may be able to see that it was the entire balancing of all the forces in our lives—good, bad, and indifferent—that have contributed to the person we are. Without a balancing of many forces, we might not have learned what we have learned and be the person we have become.

Focus on someone you believe has treated you badly and see what important lessons you have learned from that experience. You may be surprised!

SPIRITUAL BALANCE

People are equal partners with the plants and animals, not their masters who exploit them.

HAIDA GWAII

For so many centuries we have been taught that we, as people, are the highest form of evolution. This illusion has resulted in a very unbalanced planet and a lack of awareness of the interdependence and balance of all things.

Do the trees need us to grow and flourish? No, they don't! Do we need them to exist? Yes, we do. Do the rocks need us to continue to do what rocks do? No, they don't! Do we need the rocks to continue to do what we do? Yes, we do.

Oddly, it is when we begin to give up the power and responsibility of being the most important part of creation that we begin to ease into the warm bath of balance.

We have become unbalanced in the way we see the world and the place we have in it. We need to shift our perspective to greater and greater wholes in order to achieve the balance we so seek in our lives.

Ponder the idea that we need the trees and the rocks and that they don't really need us and see what happens.

PERSPECTIVE

Life comes in clusters, clusters of solitude, then a cluster when there is hardly time to breathe.

MAY SARTON

Perspective is one of the most valuable gifts we can have. Some believe that perspective can only come with age and experience. Both help. And, anyone can have perspective or not have it. One gains perspective by being able to rise above the day-to-day and see a larger picture while still participating in what is going on at the moment.

Often, we are given the gift of perspective by reading or listening to the words of people who are able to have a larger vision than we have. There's nothing wrong with not having a very large perspective. We are where we are. We are who we are.

It is a shame, however, to deprive ourselves of a broader perspective just because we don't have one ourselves. We have access to so much wisdom. There are the wise, old elders who are in our lives or who come in and out of our lives. There are the words of the great spiritual leaders. There are wonderous spiritual teachers. There are meditation books and books of wisdom.

We deprive ourselves when we do not avail ourselves of the wisdom and perspective around us. Perspective is a great balancer.

Gather some books that you know contain wisdom and perspective. Feed yourself at least once or twice a day.

DESTRUCTIVENESS

*The Great Spirit puts a shadow in your heart when you
destroy . . .*

JOE FRIDAY

We are not put here to be destructive. Whenever we are
destructive, we disturb the balance—not only our balance—we
disturb the balance that longs to exist around us.

Someone does something and we get angry about it. That's
okay. It's okay to feel angry. And, whatever that person has
done, even if it was mean and destructive, does not give us
license to behave in the same way. We have other options. We
have the option to do our own work around what was triggered
for us and then let it go. It serves no one to behave the way the
other person has behaved.

Then, there are also times when *we* do something destructive. We yell at our children, we are inattentive to those we
love, or we have a lapse in responsibility and hurt others.
When we do these things, it is our responsibility to restore the
balance. We need to do our work and, without blaming others,
take responsibility for our actions and make amends to those we
have harmed with our actions—including ourselves. We need
to set the record straight.

*At the end of the day, sit down and write down any harm
you have caused that day and see what you have to do to
restore balance.*

KNOWING THE SELF

Zen in its essence is the art of seeing into the nature of one's being, and it points the way from bondage to freedom.

D. T. SUZUKI

What difficulty we have believing that the spark of the divine infinite is within each of us and that we have the ability to link in to that spark whenever we wish. We modern people find it hard to remember that the path to the balance of living we so seek is within us, not external to us. We are so trained to look outside of ourselves for answers that we do it without missing a beat.

How important it is to take the time to go inside and explore our inner universe! We need to explore our thoughts, reactions, and feelings while participating in them fully. We need to stop when we have a reaction to a situation and see what is behind that reaction. We need to honor that reaction and ourselves. We would not have had it without a reason. What can we learn from it?

To assume that our reactions are right or wrong is to miss the point. They are neither right nor wrong. They are our schools for learning. We can always learn from our inner universe.

Today, notice your reactions and see what you can learn from them.

CONGRUENCE

Actions speak louder than words.

PROVERB

How hollow our words are when they are not supported by our actions!

Children learn at a very young age that they are safer when they respond to what their parents *do* rather than to what they *say* if the two messages differ.

For example, when someone says that she is quite open and wants to learn from us and then she interrupts and refuses to listen to anything we say, the message we get is that of her actions, not of her words.

When we say that we will follow through on our share of the housework and then don't, our partners and roommates quickly learn that they can't trust us.

Many people will promise anything in the glow of the moment and do nothing in the heat of the day.

When we behave this way, the other person (or persons) is not the greatest loser. We are. When our actions do not fit our words, not only do we set off a negative chain reaction outside ourselves, we set off a negative chain reaction within ourselves. We learn not to trust ourselves, and we feed an unbalancing process within ourselves that leads to low self-esteem and uneasiness. We cannot be dishonest with others without being dishonest to ourselves.

Set up a plan with yourself to check out the congruence or incongruence between your actions and your words, and then clean up this part of your life.

SCHEDULING

When you schedule every minute of your workday, you do not have time to put out the small fires that come up all day long. . .
Solution: Only schedule 40 to 50 percent of your day.

ROGER BROWNER

The first step to getting organized may be to take a long, hard look at who is doing the scheduling and how it is being done. Although most of us busy people tend to feel overextended and that too many demands are being made upon us, most of us do not stop to recognize that we have more control over our time than we think we do.

Somewhere along the line we came to believe that success would be achieved when we had every minute scheduled. We have come to relate full schedules to full productivity. Yet, Roger Browner, having interviewed the most successful CEOs and top business leaders, tells us that they have learned to schedule only 40 to 50 percent of their working day. What a concept! If it works for them, it might be worth trying.

Try scheduling only 40 to 50 percent of your working day and see what happens.

HUMOR

I realize that humor isn't for everyone. It's only for people who want to have fun, enjoy life, and feel alive.

ANNE WILSON SCHAEF

Choices—we all have choices. The choices we make in the little things often determine where the big ones fall.

Take humor, for example. Almost every aspect of our lives has the potential for having some humor in it. We set up a fool-proof retirement plan. We hire a good investment person, we pay costly actuaries and lawyers, and we happily plop in money for several years—only to discover that the investment person was at best incompetent, the actuary was an alcoholic, and the lawyer was a joke. Meanwhile, the IRS is panting at the door. What do we do? Slit our wrists? Cry and rage in frustration? Maybe—or we can laugh and mumble something about the "best-laid plans of mice and men" and move on into the salvage operation.

Nothing seems certain in this life except the periodic need for salvage operations.

Taking life too seriously could be a fatal disease. Of course, an old elder friend of mine reminded me recently that *"life* is a fatal disease; no one gets out of it alive."

Humor helps us have fun, enjoy life, and feel alive, even when things are not going as planned.

How often do you invite humor into your life? Every serious issue has a funny side. See if you can let yourself see it.

COMING UNGLUED

Coming unglued may mean that I am moving to a new phase of equilibrium.

ANNE

Our inner beings seem to abhor the static. Just when we think we finally have it all together and we can coast for a while, we get hit with a new kind of curveball and suddenly everything that looked like it was together is up in the air again.

Don't give up! Even though we may view being unglued as some kind of failure (a failure to be perfect, that is!), it's anything but. It's just our inner being's way of telling us that we have reached a place of awareness and strength that we are ready to move to a new level in our growth and development.

Stasis is not a normal state for the human organism, even though we would like it to be. We may get little periods in which we can rest and catch our breath and life is an ever-moving, ever-growing process. We find that when we don't fight life and join in and participate in it, life is easier. "Losing it" may be the next step.

Embrace the chaos in your life and see what happens.

MIRRORS

It is very easy to forgive others their mistakes; it takes more grit and gumption to forgive them for having witnessed your own.
JESSAMYN WEST

How we hate to be seen!

One of the most common fears we have—though it is generally voiced very carefully, if at all—is that someone will see through us or see something about us that we ourselves don't know.

We want to control how others see us and, even more so, what they see *in* us. We want to believe that we are the masters of our identity and that we do, indeed, know more about ourselves than anyone else can possibly know. Well, we have a *little bit* of the truth here.

We are *capable* of knowing more about ourselves than anyone else. And there are things we know and can know about ourselves that no one else can possibly know. *And,* we are surrounded by mirrors. People are the mirrors in our lives. One of the reasons they are there is to reflect our blind spots so we can push beyond our own limited self-knowledge and expand our learning about ourselves. We may not always like this process, and we may not always like what we see. That's okay. Both are still important.

Remember, we are mirrors for others too. Being open to this process balances it. The more we let others see us, the more we can learn about ourselves.

Take a look at the way you deal with others seeing your faults and mistakes. Is there something you need to work on here?

TENDERNESS

Tenderness is greater proof of love than the most passionate of vows.

MARLENE DIETRICH

Tenderness has a tendency to get lost in the shuffle these days, especially when we are feeling a little off-balance. We have developed a belief (probably mistaken!) that tenderness can make us vulnerable, and we are afraid of vulnerable. Nothing could be further from the truth of reality. Tenderness makes us stronger.

When we reach into tenderness in ourselves, we reach into that deep pool of our being that lets us remember ourselves as loving people. This memory is always a balancer.

At other times we may feel confused about which situations have to be handled tenderly. There is a prevalent illusion that tenderness is not strong and that we need to look strong in some situations. What a hoot! Tenderness requires greater strength, not less.

We can practice tenderness wherever we are, whenever we wish. Strength comes from the strangest places.

Take a risk in the direction of tenderness today and see what happens.

LIVING EACH AGE

I didn't fear old age. I was just becoming increasingly aware of the fact that the only people who said old age was beautiful were usually twenty-three years old.

ERMA BOMBECK

The real challenge is being the age we are!

One of the common distractions we humans use to keep our-selves unbalanced is not accepting or not being accepted as the age we are.

When we were children we were told to "grow up." We were told we were "acting like children" (which was confusing since we *were* children).

When we grew older, we were encouraged to search for the "child within" and to learn to play.

We hold the cultural belief of hoping and wanting to stay forever young.

How confusing!

Each age is different, and each is so utterly valuable. If we can live each as we do it, we will have all the ages that went before with us as we move into the next phases of our lives. We do not need to leave the ages behind; we build on them.

Why worry about old age? If we really live each age, old age will be a glorious culmination.

Sit down and let your memory gently touch the experiences of each age you have passed. Remember the fun, the struggles, and the pain. They are all yours.

LAUGHTER

Genuine laughter is the physical effect produced in the rational being by what suddenly strikes his immortal soul as being damned funny.

HILAIRE BELLOC

Have you ever been in a good restaurant and seen the other guests (not you, of course!) become annoyed when a group at one table is convulsing in laughter? In fact, how often do you see people convulsing in laughter these days? There seems to be a cultural mistrust and embarrassment with laughter, unless, of course, it is in a controlled situation. It seems that children are constantly "shushed" when they are laughing. Comics rarely win Academy Awards, and we are told that funny people are not taken seriously. Are we being conditioned to not laugh?

What fun it is to have a good laugh, one that bubbles from our pelvis right through the top of our head. I have a good friend with whom I laugh. We do many things together, and one of the most important is . . . we laugh. He calls on the phone and we start the conversation with laughter—often laughter at the sheer joy of living and being friends.

When was the last time you had a good belly laugh? Are you suppressing your laughter? Laughter is good for the body and good for the soul. Lighten up.

LISTS

I live by lists.

SUSIE

Aren't lists great? Anyone who has the courage or stupidity (or both!) to malign lists should be shot at sunrise.

Lists are one of the quickest roads back to order and sanity when life seems to spin out of control.

One of the beautiful things lists do is give us a peaceful illusion of finiteness in an infinite world. The illusion, of course, may be short-lived, and the momentary pause it gives us to get our feet back solidly on the ground may be well worth it.

Lists also feed our belief that we *can* get organized and that organization *will work.* This belief also is vital at times and will keep us stepping up to the plate.

Probably the greatest thing about lists is the sheer joy of checking items off as we do them. If we are feeling really bad, it's good to add things we have already completed to the list just so we have the pleasure of checking them off.

Feel unbalanced? Indulge in lists.

CLOSED MINDS

A closed mind is always fighting to keep everything else at arm's length.

RICHARD CARLSON

How much energy must be expended to "keep everything else at arm's length"!

If we decided we wanted to have open minds, we could let in all kinds of information. We could sort it, keeping what we like and throwing away what we don't want. And we could use what we kept to move on to bigger and better things with the same amount of energy we had been using to keep everything else out. Doesn't it seem strange that we make some of the choices we make? The logic seems so illogical.

Let's face it, a closed mind means exhaustion with little to show for it. An open mind may also be exhausting at times and at least we have something to show for our efforts. Closed minds are probably based on fear and insecurity. It's okay to be fearful and insecure. All of us are at times. It's a pity to let fear and insecurity prevent us from experiencing the glorious feast that life is offering us.

Check out the areas in which you may have a closed mind. (Most of us have some somewhere.) See if you want to make a few changes. Closed minds tip our sense of balance. Balance is most difficult with a closed mind.

BEING RIGHT

Do you prefer that you be right or happy?
A COURSE IN MIRACLES

We have a tendency to get ourselves into situations where we can develop the illusion that being right is more important than anything else in the world. As the issues escalate in our minds, we get to a place where being right seems like a life-or-death position. When we get this way, we lose all sense of perspective. We forget how important certain people are to us and what they contribute to our lives. We find ourselves more dedicated to being right than to running the risk of getting what we want, which is often happiness, love, and friendship.

What has happened to us? It seems as though we have plunged into moments of complete insanity. And, perhaps we have if insanity is related to forcing ourselves to lose perspective, lose contact with reality, and risk abandoning what is most important to us.

Are our positions more important than our happiness? Is whatever point we are trying to make more important than people we love? Very doubtful.

The next time you find yourself in this state of mind, stop. Ask yourself if you want to be right or happy. See if you really care that much. See if you can reach out—even let the other person be right. What does it really matter?

Choose very carefully the hill you want to die on and try not to sacrifice yourself on too many unimportant hills.

HATRED

The hatred of other men destroys your own soul.
SAYINGS OF THE FATHERS 2:15

How often we are able to convince ourselves that we do not really hate. Others hate. We don't. Despots hate. We don't. One has to be important or some kind of lowlife to hate. We dislike, resent, ignore, or get mad at. We don't hate.

Unfortunately, all of these "negative" emotions are branches of the same plant. Dislikes and resentments—when nurtured, fertilized, and watered, can all grow into full-blossoming trees of hatred.

When tension exists between ourselves and another, hatred is only possible if we focus our hopes, needs, and expectations outside of ourselves rather than deal with our own issues and our own pieces of the puzzle. When this kind of tension arises we have given our power away and resent the "other" for taking it.

In this situation, the only way we can get back in balance with ourselves is to stop, put the focus back on ourselves, and see what is going on with *us*. When we do this, often whatever the *real* problem is has nothing to do with the other person at all. That person is just the trigger for the opportunity to do our work and gain more clarity about our part of the situation.

Make a list of resentments you are holding on to and see what you need to do with yourself to feel better.

THE WEATHER

I don't like it that I am affected by the weather.

JULIUS

So!? We *are* affected by the weather, you know. Regardless of how hard we try to build artificial climates in our homes, offices, and shopping centers, we are still affected by changes in the weather. Sunny days affect us differently than rainy days and when we have too many hot, sunny days, we begin to long for a quiet, rainy day to give us relief.

The beauty of our being affected by the weather is that we can have an ever-so-slight awareness that we are a part of something much larger than ourselves. Even if we are not aware of our full participation, our body's response to the weather can give us a glimpse of being a part of a much bigger whole and participating with it.

Our responsibility is to participate with the weather around us. The weather may be offering us just what we need. We may begrudge a snow day, yet a quiet day at home may be just what the doctor ordered. A sunny day may beckon us to come out into the air. When we live *with* the weather, our lives feel more balanced.

Take a look at the way you respond to the weather. If you think you're in control, take a closer look.

TOSS, REFER, ACT, OR FILE

Executive coach, bestselling author, and noted executive organizer Stephanie Winston has come up with a simple and enormously effective way to tame the paper tiger. She has named it TRAF, which stands for Toss, Refer, Act, or File!

ROGER BROWNER

TRAF—it sounds so simple, doesn't it? Let's work backward: *File.* For many of us, there is very little that comes in the mail that we really want to file. To warrant filing, it needs to be important now or possibly important later, requiring no immediate action.

Action. Does something need to be done with this? If so, do whatever can be done immediately or put it in a file or pile to be handled as soon as feasible. Immediate action is the best.

Refer. Some things are just none of our business, can be better handled by others, or we just don't want to take care of them. Then, pass them on, *immediately.* We don't have to control or do everything, whether we are in the office or at home. Learn to pass information, requests, ideas, and tasks along—immediately! What a relief.

Toss. Here's the hard one. What if we might want this later? Maybe we could take time to read it more thoroughly later (when?). There *might* be something of interest we *may* need to know. Trust your first impulse and toss it.

Put a large wastebasket near where the mail or papers are collected and/or sorted.

GOING INTO THE SILENCE

Their [The American Indians] favorite method for acquiring fresh wisdom and knowledge, and especially immediately needed information, was not to seek it vocally from some other Indian or even from printed words. On the contrary, each individually went into the silence, with his silence and then let the silence whisper to him whatever it was that he specifically needed to know. . . . the silence had never once failed to cooperate with them in this manner.

J. ALLEN BOONE

There is such peace in going into the silence!

The Quakers call it the "inner light."

It is such an act of faith to believe that all the information we need can come through us and be available inside of us if we only have the willingness and the patience to learn how to "wait with" the silence.

Waiting with the silence is an active place of quiet, a quiet place of action. Waiting with is not passive. Nor is it demanding. Moving into the silence requires that we shed all expectations while knowing that our answers are there. It is a place beyond thinking and reasoning, a place of silent, open anticipation. The information in that quiet place is the information and wisdom of the all that is, and it is available to us if we are available to it.

We do not need meditation techniques and positions to enter the silence, only the desire to do so. Give yourself opportunities for going into the silence every day. You'll not regret it.

WORKAHOLISM

I'm beginning to question whether workaholism is worth it.
CHARLES

Aren't we great?! We participate in behaviors that we know are destructive to ourselves and others. We run ourselves ragged. We threaten our health. We alienate those who love us the most. We do this all for power and money, or so we believe! And then one day we wake up and *start* to question whether all this stress is worth it.

Who do we think we are—stand-up comics? What a routine! It's as if we have suddenly become a master of the obvious and we would like others to believe that we have discovered the secret to the universe and we want others to recognize the corner on wisdom we have just flagged.

Relax. Many other workaholics and people who do too much have come to the same realization and nothing has changed.

It's the action that counts.

Try getting yourself to a Workaholics Anonymous meeting or setting up a regular appointment to examine your overdoing with another workaholic friend (if you can find the time!).

COOPERATION

The only thing that will redeem mankind is cooperation.
BERTRAND RUSSELL

Competition is such a given in our way of life that we rarely stop to realize that without cooperation, competition would not be possible. We tend to mask the cooperation that is the foundation of all that exists, focusing instead on competition. We focus on competition to such an extent that cooperation gets lost in the shuffle.

Being a star athlete is great. Yet, would it be possible without a team? And, if we are not talking about a team sport, could a Tiger Woods be a Tiger Woods without coaches, parents, teachers, manufacturers of equipment, and the gardeners and personnel who manicure the golf courses?

Whatever we accomplish or will accomplish is because at some level in our lives and in the lives that preceded ours there was a level of cooperation that made whatever exists today and whoever we are today possible.

When we realize that we can act, and indeed we do, and each action is always in cooperation with the seen and the unseen, we gain more perspective on ourselves and on life.

Today (and every day), be aware of how what you do and are doing is grounded in cooperation.

COMPASSION

Spiritual energy brings compassion into the real world. With compassion, we see benevolently our own human condition and the condition of our fellow beings. We drop prejudice. We withhold judgment.

CHRISTINA BALDWIN

We are all blessed with spiritual energy. To be human in its fullest sense means that we are spiritual, and our spirits possess an energy that is both compassionate and healing. We are not gods and we are also much more divine than we allow ourselves to recognize. Divinity and humanness are our birthrights. It's the living out of all these potentials that sometimes offers us a challenge.

When we see ourselves as we truly are—divinely perfect human beings struggling to live out the gifts of spirituality—we have an opportunity to crack open the door of compassion a bit. When we can compassionately see that we fumble, we make mistakes, or that we are (if only faintly and occasionally!) aware of a goodness within us that we do not always know how to express, we start to be aware of feelings of compassion for ourselves. Once we are aware of compassion for ourselves, it is only a very short step to begin to feel compassion for others.

Practice forgiving yourself for being human. Then, pass that forgiveness on to others.

WHOLEHEARTEDNESS

The most comprehensive formulation of therapeutic goals is striving for wholeheartedness: *to be without pretense, to be emotionally sincere, to be able to put the whole of oneself into one's feelings, one's work, one's beliefs.*

KAREN HORNEY

To be without pretense is a necessity for feeling balanced and whole. Pretending we are who we are not always lends an element of fear to our lives.

When we are pretending to be something or someone we are not, we cannot help but feel uneasy. We are always having to look over our shoulders lest we be found out. Sometimes, we fear that if we become too good at pretending, we, ourselves, will be fooled and will forget who we really are. Then, there is always the uneasiness of not knowing if our friends like us because of who they *think* we are or because of who we really are. The longer we pretend, the more difficult it is for us to break the pattern.

Why do we have such a problem with the simplicity of just being who we are? We may be "unusual," slightly odd, or even very creative. The important issue is that we are perfectly unique. There never has been and never will be anyone like us. We are a one-time creation and can add much more to the world when we are wholeheartedly ourselves. The world needs our unique contributions.

How would your life change if you jumped into every aspect of it wholeheartedly being yourself? See if there are some changes you want to make. Try an idea that is wholly you and see where you can go with it.

STRUGGLING

Strugglers like to feel that struggle is noble—that somehow God is pleased with them for struggling. If you were God, you would fall over laughing at that one.

STUART WILDE

Ah, the nobility of struggling! Are you a struggler? Do you see yourself as a struggler? Are you one of those people who believe that life is hard and that anything that comes easily to you must be suspect?

Take another look.

Are you actually contributing to the struggling by believing in struggle? We can do that, you know. Belief is a very powerful motivator *and* determiner of events. Thinking doesn't exactly make it so and it goes a long way as a contributor to struggling. I have known people with very difficult lives who don't struggle, and I have known people with lives that could be very easy who make a struggle out of everything. The choice is ours.

> When you find yourself struggling, stop to determine whether you are contributing to the struggle. What is your attitude? What could you do differently? How is your attitude toward struggle related to your attempt to control people, persons, things, and events over which you have no control? See what happens if you give up struggling and simply approach the issue as a task or situation to be dealt with.

KNOWING GOD

Never trust someone who has to change his tone to ask something of the Lord.

ROBERTA A. EVERETT

What good advice! If God is everywhere, why can't we whisper? Or why talk at all? Surely God is telepathic.

I can remember as a child that I never trusted ministers who changed their voice to talk with God. I always wondered if God was hard of hearing, because the volume went up. I can remember thinking that I would hate to be yelled at that way, in a rather unctuous, unnatural voice.

I wonder how much of our resistance to and confusion about God is related to our experience of the "authorities" on God we knew as children.

God is mysterious and beyond our knowing and there is no mystery about God if *we* don't make our knowing too complex.

Study a flower and know God. Watch a child and know God. Feel love in your chest and know God. Rejoice in your sexuality and know God. Enjoy the feel of water on your body and know God. Experience the comfort in the coming of each new day and know God. Have a brilliant new idea and know God. Solve a problem and know God. It's all quite simple. Don't think too much.

WORK AS MEDITATION

Let us work without theorizing; it is the only way to make life endurable.

VOLTAIRE

What a joy it is when we can just participate in our work without thinking about it too much. Our full participation has a way of freeing the soul. Our theorizing, on the other hand, has a way of removing us from ourselves and our task, resulting in both ourselves and our task becoming abstractions.

How simple our work becomes when we become one with it!

I have come to believe that Westerners have a constitutional difficulty with meditation. It is very hard for us to sit, clear our minds, and move beyond ourselves. Yet, I believe that almost every person has found a way of meditation that fits for them. Some mow the grass; others wash the dishes; others polish the car; some refinish furniture; some fold laundry; others take walks. Meditation is whatever we can do where we fully participate and experience mindlessness.

Our lives move into balance when we find our own personal ways of meditation. Perhaps the "meaningless tasks" have more meaning than we ever realized!

What is your meditative work process? Do it!

HABITS

We are what we repeatedly do. Excellence, then is not an act, but a habit.

ARISTOTLE

Rarely do we stop to take a close look at the habits we have built during our lives. Yet, these habits have much more influence over us than we would like to admit.

Over the years, some of us have developed the habit of speeding. We are not *really* speeders like those BMWs, Porsches, or Mercedes, that fly by us on the throughway. We are careful, thoughtful speeders. We go just a little bit over the speed limit, usually, we hope, just enough not to get caught and yet enough that we can make a little better time than if we stuck to the speed limit. We are living on the edge, honey. We do not generate huge amounts of adrenaline, we only generate just enough to keep us a little high. We are indulging in a habit that stresses our bodies and keeps us looking over our shoulder. Do we need this? Probably not. Does it interfere with habits of excellence we could form in its place? Probably.

Or, have we developed a habit of doing as much as we can at the last minute, then marveling at what a good job we did under pressure? Does this have the same effect on our minds, bodies, and souls as speeding just a little? Probably.

The lovely fact about habits is that they can be changed. We built them. We can dismantle them.

Take a look at the subtle habits that are eroding your life. What habits of excellence could you replace them with?

HECKLING

Tommy Trinder gave me invaluable advice about hecklers. "Always get them to repeat what they have said," he told me, "because nothing sounds quite so funny or offensive when it is repeated."

MICHAEL BENTINE

What good advice!

There are very few of us who do anything at all who manage to get through life without being harassed by hecklers at some point. The problem with hecklers is not the hecklers themselves. They are a given in life, and ultimately they have to deal with themselves. The biggest problem with hecklers is what *we* do with them. We imbue them with truth, power, and intelligence—all of which may very well be lacking or they would not choose to waste their time being hecklers and would get on with their own lives.

What exactly do I mean by hecklers? Hecklers are people who try to undermine everything we do, especially if we are doing it well and are successful at it. Who are our hecklers? Well, I hate to say it and our worst hecklers tend to be ourselves. We lie in wait with ourselves, watching for what could be a mistake, and then we let fly with a barrage of thoughts or mumblings that would stop a charging cavalry. Others may try similar techniques with us and the one who has the most damning information and is the most dangerous is ourself.

When your heckler sounds off inside your head, repeat it to a good friend and have a good laugh together.

HOME ALONE

Be able to be alone. Lose not the advantage of solitude.
SIR THOMAS BROWNE

It is absolutely essential to be in our homes with no one else around sometimes. Whether we live with only ourselves or live with a house full of people, there are times when we vitally need to be in and with our homes alone.

When the last person walks out and closes the door, we and the house simultaneously heave an audible sigh. There is something about being home alone that allows us to move slowly through the house, preparing to gather the far-flung pieces of ourselves that have become distributed elsewhere while we were "doing" our lives.

Being home alone allows us to pull ourselves into ourselves and snuggle down in a known and loved environment to regroup and prepare to participate in the active aspects of our lives.

Supreme luxury would be having a whole day at home with ourselves once in a while. Still, never underestimate what even an hour alone with a good cup of tea can do to return us to balance.

There is no quiet like the quiet of being alone with oneself at home.

Arrange for some alone time at home sometime soon and allow yourself to regroup.

CHILDREN—ENCHANTMENT— VALIDATION

Parents of young children should realize that few people, and maybe no one, will find their children as enchanting as they do.

BARBARA WALTERS

We can throw ourselves completely off balance wanting others to validate the deep enchantment we feel for our children. Who needs it? We really do not need another's validation for feelings we have, no matter what the feelings are. And, when we get right down to it, the real truth is that nobody can validate another person or what she or he feels anyway. True validation can only come from within, and no human being possesses the right or the ability to validate another. When we seek validation for our feelings from others, we are giving our power away by the bucketload and asking for something that is not possible, creating a huge imbalance in our life.

That said, let's take the magical opportunity to be completely enchanted by our children or, if we have no children, by other people's children. The wonderful thing about children is that they can quite easily and with no apparent negative side effects absorb all the enchanted words, feelings, and looks adults can heap upon them. The exciting thing is that when adults let themselves become enchanted by anything—especially a baby or a child—they become more lovable themselves.

See if you can indulge in some enchantment this week—with a child would be a nice touch.

LOVE

Love is like a baby: it needs to be treated tenderly.

ZAIREAN PROVERB

All too rarely do we stop to let ourselves realize what a gift love is. We get so bound up in our expectations, wants, and needs that we lose track of what is being given to us.

How lucky we are to experience the love of animals! What a tender, sweet gift is the dog who unconditionally meets us at the door with tail wagging, the cat who conditionally allows us to be her friend, or the horse who patiently waits for the next contact, nickering as we approach!

How honored we are when children choose to love us and give us their trust. The love of a child is such a precious, gentle gift. We have a great responsibility to treat it tenderly.

Have we treated the love of our parents tenderly? Even if they did not meet our expectations or the cultural norm of loving, have we been able to see that, given who they are and their experiences, they have done the best they could with what they had?

Are we open to being tender with love whenever and wherever it finds us?

What ways can you improve your tenderness with love?

FOOLING OURSELVES

Telling ourselves it ain't so doesn't make it not so.

ELOISE

We tell ourselves so many "stories" about our working too much!

"I love my work. If I were a workaholic, would I love my work?" "I'm not a workaholic. I just love to work." "I can't trust anyone else to do it right. At least if I do it myself, I know it's done right." "If I don't do it, who will?" "I don't work *all* the time." "Can anything that gives you pleasure be bad for you?" . . . And so it goes.

When we deceive ourselves, it's not a very big leap into believing that we can deceive others. As a member of the human species, we have an unfailing ability to trick ourselves into believing the most outrageous stories, stories we tell ourselves and then parade as truth. Our excuses for our acts of self-destruction are very creative, if not believable. Often, we are the only ones fooled, and the cost to our inner beings is indeed great.

Today, keep a notepad handy and try to jot down a few of the whoppers you tell yourself. Others may not even hear them, and, we do.

OPPORTUNITIES

I had to make my own living and my own opportunity . . . Don't sit down and wait for the opportunities to come; you have to get up and make them.

MADAME C. J. WALKER

"Making opportunities" may be little more than having the presence of mind to notice that they are there.

We are always surrounded by doors of opportunity. That's the way life is. Often, opportunities do not come in packages nor all wrapped in the colors we expected. When an unexpected surprise happens, we refuse to see it and so we miss the opportunity. Sometimes we are so focused on a goal far out in the future that we do not see what is right in front of us, or we get so busy hurrying and rushing around that we lose all perspective.

Opportunity can be subtle. It may be the ache or pain in our body that whispers for us to slow down before it roars. And then, when we slow down we become aware of the preciousness of what we have. Opportunity may involve taking on the task we really did not want to do and then finding that we have a knack for it. Opportunity may require trusting the "crazy" idea that shoots into our heads from nowhere that just might work. Opportunity has a lot to do with noticing.

Be aware of some of the opportunities that are presented to you this day that you might not have previously noticed and follow up on one or two.

ONENESS

From Wakan Tanka, the Great Spirit, there came a great unifying life force that flowed in and through all things—the flowers of the plains, blowing winds, rocks, trees, birds, animals—and was the same force that had been breathed into the first man. Thus all things were kindred, and were brought together by the same Great Mystery.

CHIEF LUTHER STANDING BEAR

Our Native American Indian brothers and sisters say that they were put on this earth to remember and perpetuate the basic spiritual truths so that those truths could be handed down when the world was ready to hear them. And, that time is now. There is no more basic truth than the interconnectedness of all things. It takes some time to grasp the full meaning that all creation is one—that the same force that created human beings created the rocks, the animals, and the trees. The enormity of this truth cannot be taken lightly, nor does it come easily.

To know that I am intimately connected with all that exists is both an immense relief and a huge responsibility. It is a relief to know that I am not in this life alone, that I am connected with and supported by all creation. And, if I truly *know* this connection, I am also responsible for and need to respond to all creation. Knowing these essential truths adds a balance to our lives like nothing else can.

Today, ponder and know a connection that you feel with a pet, a tree, or with the stars. Open yourself to oneness.

PEACE

In dwelling, be close to the land. In meditation go deep in the heart. In dealing with others, be gentle and kind.

LAO-TZU

How peaceful the above quote is! In only three little sentences calm is brought into our lives. What a rare and magnificent gift is peacefulness! How can we possibly expect peace on the planet if we do not know peace within ourselves?

In dwelling, be close to the land. How can we do this when our world is becoming covered with asphalt and concrete and we live on the fifteenth floor of a high-rise? Being close to the land is not easy in some situations, and it is possible in all situations. No matter what our buildings are, they are rooted in the earth. Their foundations reach into the earth and depend upon the land for their very existence. We can let the peaceful awareness of our roots reaching deep into the earth permeate our being.

In meditation, go deep in the heart. Meditation is not a head thing. The purpose of meditation is to move us beyond our busy heads into the quiet of our beings, which through our hearts connects us with the stillness of *all* being.

In dealing with others, be kind and gentle. For many of us, kindness and gentleness are learned skills. We may not have grown up with them and the exciting news is they can be learned. Since life is about learning what we have thus far missed, why not have a go at it?

Practice being close to the land, going deep in the heart, and being kind and gentle. Peace and balance are by-products of these activities.

BEING UNDERSTOOD

When my husband doesn't understand me, I can stop to see if I understand him. This is something I can do.

BETTY

We cannot *make* another person understand us. We can give information, we can share our feelings, and we can want to be understood. Yet, understanding is always at the behest of the other person; we have no control over it.

What we *can* do is shift our attention and see if we can understand the person by whom we want to be understood. We can develop an attitude of listening—not only with our ears, which is important, but with our hearts and beings. We can take in the information and let it sink into us. We can not interrupt. We can resist the temptation to assume that we know more about that person than they know about themselves. We can absolutely under no circumstances indulge in the seductive behaviors of interpreting that person. We can put all our wanting-to-be-understood energy into seeking to understand.

We may never be understood by that person and one thing is definite—we'll feel better about ourselves and more in balance.

When you find yourself in a position of wanting to be understood, shift to trying to understand. It's amazing what this shift in perspective will do.

ARGUING

I don't have to attend every argument I'm invited to.
ANONYMOUS

Some of us grew up in households where a good argument was seen as the flavoring of the day. We didn't mean anything by it. Bickering among the kids, between the kids and parents, and between and among adults was just the order of the day. Many of us grew up with the mistaken notion that fighting was a key method of establishing intimacy. Some households argue with shouts, words, and screams, while others argue with silence. Both can be devastating.

We will find that there are people in our lives who do not know how to explore an issue without presenting one opening gambit after another, turning every discussion into an argument. We have the choice as to whether we make the second move, accepting the challenge for the argument *and* this way of relating can get exhausting.

We can remember that for an argument to happen with us, we have to be willing to accept the invitation.

Setting up an argument is a lose-lose situation. Accepting the invitation to argue is a lose-lose situation. We have other options.

Develop your skills to recognize the invitation to an argument. Then, you have the choice of whether you want to participate or not.

EATING

I feel now that gastronomical perfection can be reached in these combinations: one person dining alone, usually upon a couch or a hillside; two people, of no matter what sex or age, dining in a good restaurant; six people, of no matter what sex or age, dining in a good home.

M. F. K. FISHER

Eating can be one of the ways that we return to and maintain balance.

I'm not talking about balanced and regular meals, the importance of which goes without saying. I am talking about the *process* of eating as a balancing process.

I have been eating a nutritionally balanced diet for a while and really love it. The other day I had a breakfast of cottage cheese, strawberries, pears (Harry & David—delicious!), blueberries, and nuts. I was eating slowly, savoring each taste and combination of tastes. I was aware that the blueberries, strawberries, and cottage cheese tasted different from the strawberries, pears, and cottage cheese. I savored the crunchiness of the nuts among the other, "softer" foods. I tasted each texture and flavor. I enjoyed each texture and flavor. I did nothing but eat.

When I finished, I was aware of feeling peaceful.

Try eating several (or at least one!) meals alone each week in silence—no radio, no conversation, no telephone calls, no TV, no rushing or thinking—just you, tasting the food— and see what happens. Give this more than one trial. I recommend several to allow you to settle down into the process and experience the full effect.

TIME

He (Kosirev) devised brilliant experiments that enabled him to develop a complex theory of time, proving that time has a substantial nature. It has its own solidity, which changes according to the configuration of the globe. Consequently, time is more solid or less solid at different points on the earth.

OLGA KHARITIDI

I had a friend once who told me that someday he was going to take me into the middle of Australia, where I would experience time as a substance. I have not gone there yet and I believe I have learned more about the fluidity and complexity of time in the intervening years.

Perhaps someday I will be ready to go. I have learned that time is not the hands on the clock. And I have learned that time is not linear.

Perhaps the real issue is not time itself. The issue is what we do with time.

When we try to control time or let it control us, we are probably in an unbalanced relationship with it. When we believe that we have invented time and that we understand it, we are probably confused about it. When we believe that time is the hands on the clock, we are the slave of it and seek to enslave it.

Time and space are our cutting edges. When we participate with them and do not try to control them, our boundaries expand.

Observe how time expands and contracts according to what you are doing. See if you have any influence in this process.

OUR SIMPLE COMPLEXITY

Of the doctor, the poet, and the fool we all have a small portion.
MEXICAN PROVERB

Let's not try to make ourselves too simple. We are very complex beings, and living in balance demands that we embrace that complexity even when it means contradictions within ourselves. The truth is that we human beings are a paradox: we are amazingly simple we are profoundly complex. We are much more comfortable with the simplicity and all too often try to reduce ourselves down to what we perceive to be manageable pieces. Then, to confound the picture, we discover that we are not only composed of all kinds of cooperating, conflicting, and confusing pieces, we are also made up of differing, debilitating, dramatic, and engaging and disengaging processes. What's a person to do? No wonder our first reaction is to try to reduce all this teeming mass down to a few manageable pieces. Fortunately, this strategy doesn't work. We are much too much for ourselves.

We are the doctor, the poet, and the fool, as well as the parent, the teacher, the pupil, the boss, and the employee. We are building, destroying, creating, inventing, relaxing, and plunging up, down, and sideways. We have parts of the whole, and we are the whole. Isn't this exciting?

See if there are ways you have tried to reduce yourself to a controllable size. What ways do you curb yourself in and reduce yourself? See if you really want to do this.

SELF-ACCEPTANCE

To love oneself is the beginning of a lifelong romance.
OSCAR WILDE

What person other than ourselves can we be sure will be with us from the moment of conception until the last breath leaves our body? None that I can think of. We may look for a love to be with us always and even the love of our life will not have the same duration with ourselves that we do. Let's face it: if we are looking for longevity in our relationships, we're it! That's just the way it is.

Now that we have established the point of unique longevity, let's explore some of the factors that may *limit* our romance with ourselves. This is the easiest love affair of our lives and we don't want to miss it.

Self-acceptance—now there's a tough one. Some of us are so busy trying to be someone else—who we think we should be, who society or our family thinks we should be, or who we dream we are—that we have difficulty seeing and accepting who we are at this point in time and space. The irony is that the minute we accept ourselves as we are, we can change and grow and move on.

Admitting our mistakes is one of the wide avenues leading to self-love. When we admit our mistakes and make amends for them, we reclaim our power and actually like ourselves better.

Remember, lifelong romances take time.

What do you have difficulty accepting in yourself? Take a look at what you need to do to be more forgiving of yourself.

PUSHING OURSELVES

I just can't do anymore!

RENÉ

Who said that? Every person whose life is out of balance is overcome by that feeling at some point. Yet, if we really drive ourselves, we discover that we can push our limits to the max.

We live in a culture where pushing beyond our limits and almost killing ourselves at our own expense and that of those who love us has become heroic. What a crock!

What's the joy and excitement in being "financially well taken care of" if the person who does the caring (whom we love) is a near-dead, limit-pushing hero?

There is a great difference between challenging ourselves and pushing ourselves to break our limits and ourselves.

Challenging ourselves is respectful of ourselves and others. Challenging ourselves is not a frenzied plunge to find our spirituality; it is a tender *working with* our spirituality.

Where are you pushing your limits? See if you can find your spirituality in it anywhere.

INTERRUPTIONS

Katherine Graham, CEO of the Washington Post Company, (to avoid interruptions) prefers to "pay visits" to those who work for her.

ROGER BROWNER

Browner, who writes for executive newsletters, points out that by taking the initiative to go visit her employees, Graham "has an opportunity to gather firsthand information and build strong, more personal relationships with those on her staff." "This interactive management style helps prevent the onslaught of interruptions."

When we are focused on a task, most of us abhor interruptions. We almost always see interruptions as personal and disrespectful. If we don't see them this way (or won't admit this to ourselves), we see them, at best, as bothersome.

Have we ever looked at what we can do to prevent interruptions or at how we contribute to them?

For example, a manager who does not want to be interrupted yet talks or barks orders to her staff through her open door invites interruptions. A father who does not explain that he needs some time and space, that is, until he blows up invites interruptions.

When we make it clear that we do not want to be interrupted before we start a task, we have a better chance of having our request respected.

Get some DO NOT DISTURB signs to hang on the door. Many hotels and motels will be happy to gift you with some.

SILENT, ALONE TIME

All of humanity's problems stem from man's inability to sit quietly in a room alone.

PASCAL

Have you tried sitting quietly in a room all alone lately—no television, no radio, no telephone, no welcome interruption from family or friends?

We have a basic human need for silence with ourselves. This "alone silence" is not a luxury; it is a necessity.

Pascal may be right that all of humanity's problems stem from this inability, *and* we will probably never be in a situation to prove it.

What we *are* able to do is to take the one person of ourselves and give it a try. We do not have to do anything. We do not have to say anything. We do not have to have a technique, method, or practice to distract ourselves. It is enough to sit with and wait with the silence in our aloneness and let it speak to us. It, of course, will only speak clearly when the chatter in our heads has subsided somewhat.

Try indulging in your need for silent alone time, even if you don't know that you need it.

INDIVIDUALITY AND
WHOLENESS

In this culture, at least, it seems like we never forget that we're individuals, but we're constantly forgetting that we are all one.

LIA

Those deadly dualisms! Either we are individuals or we are part of a whole. When we see the world in dualisms, we topple from one extreme to the other, never able to grasp reality.

We are individuals who exist as a part of a whole. Our individual identity is fulfilled only when we see ourselves in context. When we as individuals try to dislodge ourselves from that context, we destroy the very context we need for growth and survival. This is what we are doing to the earth right now.

When we see ourselves only as context, we ignore and devalue the absolute wonder, richness, and necessity of diversity. Our emphasis on individuality has framed itself so that only certain human individuality is important, thus making it acceptable to destroy other, "less important," aspects of the whole.

To restore balance to ourselves and our planet, we need to relearn that we are individuals, along with many other individuals—plants, animals, trees, and bugs—that are part of a larger whole on which we are all dependent.

Practice seeing yourself as an individual and as a part of a very diverse whole. When you see a bug, a tree, a plant, or another human being, let the knowledge seep into your awareness that you need that being.

ACCIDENTS

Accident is veiled necessity.

MARIE VON EBNER-ESCHENBACH

We often hear that there are no accidents. Yet unfortunate things *do* happen.

There are three important aspects of accidents that we need to consider.

First, when accidents happen, we need to accept them. They happened. We have to deal with them. That's the reality. If we choose to rant against the accidents, indulge in believing that we feel like victims, or resent them and refuse to deal with them, we only hurt ourselves. We have better things to do with our time.

Secondly, accidents often "happen" when we are off-balance, and they definitely put us off-balance. Accidents may just be a red flag that we are pushing too hard or are not present to our lives. We can see them as a signal that we need to take stock.

Lastly, we have the opportunity to turn accidents into experiences for learning. We need to see what we can learn. We need to explore *what* the "learning" is for us. Whether the accident happened to us or to someone else, there is a learning there for us. There is *always* a learning there for us—no matter what.

The next time an accident enters your life, remember the ABL of accidents—Acceptance, Balance, and Learning.

COMPASSION

The love of our neighbor in all its fullness simply means being able to say to him, "What are you going through?"

SIMONE WEIL

For some of us, "loving our neighbor as ourselves" is a big order, especially if we are critical of ourselves. Of course, if we are hypercritical of ourselves, there is no way we are not going to be critical and judgmental of others.

One of the positions we human beings take is, "If I can't do it all, I won't do anything."

Let's back off from the whole, big, seemingly impossible mandate of being a "compassionate person" and take some little steps. Are we able to say to our neighbor, our boss, our friend, our spouse, our children, "What are you going through?"— and then listen to the response to our question? If we can, compassion practice is paying off.

Practice being truly concerned about what others are going through even when you don't know what to do or can do nothing. You won't be sorry.

WEAKNESS—HIGHER POWER

. . . it is precisely the weakness in whatever goodness we do have a share in that gives us our claim on reality and on the help of a Higher Power.

ERNEST KURTZ AND KATHERINE KETCHAM

Admitting the importance of our weaknesses is not always easy. Yet our weakness is one of our most important avenues to balance.

This may come as a shock to some of you, but we are human beings. We all have the spark of the Divine within us, *and* we are first and most completely human beings.

Human beings make mistakes. We do wrong things. We get in trouble. That's just the way it is, and we can see these "weaknesses" as our greatest opportunities for learning, which they are. These "defects" are the very things we need to help us see reality. Only when we see reality can we know that we really do not run the whole shebang, nor are we responsible for it all. We are only responsible for our little piece and our individual behaviors. We simply do not have what it takes to be responsible for it all. "It" is much bigger than our imaginations or reality.

Seeing and accepting our weakness develops humility. Humility allows us genuinely to ask for help. For some of us, it takes a while to believe that we have a Higher Power willing to help.

Daily, allow yourself to be open to the positive importance of any weakness and test out asking a Higher Power for help. See what happens.

LOSS OF ILLUSIONS

Our losses include not only our separations and departures from those we love, but our conscious and unconscious losses of romantic dreams, impossible expectations, illusions of freedom and power, illusions of safety—and the loss of our own younger self, the self that thought it would always be unwrinkled and invulnerable and immortal.

JUDITH VIORST

Why is it that we always tend to think of losses as negative and resulting in our having less? This perception probably relates to our trying to control our lives rather than participating in them, as well as our trying to make the living, moving process that is life's reality static.

Take romantic dreams for example. Have we ever stopped to realize how much trouble our romantic dreams get us into? When we insist on our romantic notions, we absolutely refuse to see people and life the way they are and try every means possible to *make the situation the way we want it.* We cling to who we *want* people to be, refusing to get to *know* them. What a loss! We may be grieving the wrong thing. When we grieve loss, what we may really need to grieve is the loss of knowing the real person, not our fantasy of them.

Many people find that losing their romantic dreams and impossible expectations is a *relief.* It's like a heavy backpack we have been lugging around has been put to rest.

Maybe, just maybe, when we change our attitude toward losses, we will have more energy to live life.

Are you clinging to some fond illusions that you are ready to leave behind? Take a look.

OUR BODIES

Bodies never lie.

AGNES DE MILLE

Learning to live in balance means learning to listen to our bodies. Bodies are not just a mechanical structure we live in for a while and then discard. They are much, much more than that.

Our bodies are sophisticated, subtle, intricate, wondrous combinations of activities, electrical impulses, and living processes; they are storers of memories, receivers, processors, gatherers, and transmitters of information, tellers of the way we are living our lives, registerers of stress and strain, warning bells when we are getting into trouble, and providers of pleasure and joy and all of the range of emotions we feel and can feel as human beings. We have barely tapped into all the wonders our bodies can accomplish, and I'm not talking about pushing the envelope to see how far we can go and how much we can take.

Our bodies are there for us. Are we there for them?

When our bodies tell us they need rest, solitude, time out, exercise, good food, or healing, do we listen? If we are listening, they will never lie. Even if we're *not* listening, they will never lie.

What does your body need right now? Shut off that thinking and listen. Can and will you respond?

PRAYER—PATIENCE

The greatest prayer is patience.

GAUTAMA BUDDHA

"I'm a very patient person," you say—perhaps like Dustin Hoffman's character in *Rain Man*, who kept repeating, "I'm an excellent driver!"

Patience is one of those slippery concepts that sounds good and is definitely more positive in other people.

Why should we be patient? We have too many, too important things to do. Patience is for the elderly, or at least for the middle-aged, who have begun to slow down. And, we're not ready to slow down yet. Right? Wrong! Patience is important at *all* ages.

What is patience?

Patience is an act of faith—of *great* faith—that life is as it is, that at some ultimate level, everything is as it should be and will unfold as it will.

Patience is the ability to "wait with." Waiting *with* is much different than waiting *for*. When we wait *for*, we still indulge in the illusion that we are ultimately in control.

Patience is the curiosity of belief. It is the openness to adventure into the unknown, a readiness to be surprised.

Patience is serenity in the face of insanity. It is *not* white-knuckled control.

Where do you stand in relation to patience? Is this one of your cutting edges? Patience is a learned skill and can be learned by any motivated person. Pray for the willingness to be patient.

HIGHER LEARNING

I don't know what is better than the work that is given to the actor—to teach the human heart the knowledge of itself.

LAURENCE OLIVIER

We are all actors. Our stages may be different and our audiences may be only ourselves, yet, a major role we have in life is to teach our human heart (and maybe even others!) the knowledge of ourself.

Knowledge of the self brings a freedom to be, to act, to know, and to soar and connect beyond ourselves.

Ignorance of ourselves can be celebrated only in the potential for learning about ourselves. Without knowledge of ourselves, we act and react in knee-jerk fashion, leaving the devastations of these actions and reactions for others to deal with and clean up.

Within each of us is a universe of learning. Unfortunately, despite our modern techniques, this universal university cannot be accessed through our conscious mind. We need to access the higher school of learning through our bodies and our feelings— through our hearts. Only then can we bring the knowledge to our brains to be sorted and named.

Once we have experienced conscious living, we will never want to return to emotional ignorance.

Have you seen or read a good play recently? Plays help to access our centers of higher learning. Try it.

REGRETS—COURAGE

Regrets are as personal as fingerprints.
MARGARET CULKIN BANNING

My regrets are mine. Whatever I have done to cause regret, I did it myself. I may have been pushed by others and circumstances may have prodded me hard. Yet, when all is said and done, I am the one who acted or did not act, and that is my reality.

Often, we keep our lives in imbalance by trying to blame others for our actions and decisions. There are as many forms of "He/she/they made me do it" as there are stars in the sky.

Unfortunately, what we fail to realize in the "others made me do" stance is that in this process we give our power away by the truckload and then bemoan that we feel put upon.

It takes courage to own our behaviors and take responsibility for our actions. It takes courage to stand up and say that we made the decision and we regret it. It takes courage to admit to our personal regrets and own them as fully as we can. Yet, when we do, the door to personal freedom and power is suddenly before us.

Take a month to remember and list some personal regrets that you carry. Then go over them with someone you trust to see what you need to do about them.

SIMPLIFY

The ability to simplify means to eliminate the unnecessary so that the necessary may speak.

HANS HOFMANN

Often when we think of simplifying our lives, the image that comes to our minds is one of giving up, having less, or suffering. We immediately jump to the "natural" conclusion that to simplify means to live in a cave somewhere without heat or electricity, probably wearing a loincloth. Aren't our minds funny? That image is disturbing enough to keep us safely away from any notion of simplifying for some time to come, trusting that if we ever do approach the concept again, our active minds will again rescue us. Let's hear it for negative thinking!

Now, just for fun, let's approach the idea of simplifying from a positive perspective. What if we actively choose to simplify "to eliminate the unnecessary so that the necessary can speak." Clutter is a fact of modern living. We have cluttered drawers, cluttered closets, cluttered garages, cluttered schedules, and, all too often, cluttered lives. In such cluttered lives, do we really have room for the necessary to speak? Is the important hidden by the unimportant? Do our "necessaries" change as we change, and then we forget to discard the "unnecessaries"? Have we deprived ourselves of the voice of the necessary?

If you are willing to enter upon an experiment, make a commitment to eliminate one "unnecessary" from your life each week for a year and see how you feel.

EATING

You may not know it, but Scotch tape holds a meat loaf together beautifully. I always use it if I'm out of Band-Aids or rubber bands. A little ketchup will cover up the flavor. Before I did this, I could never slice a meat loaf—it exploded.

PHYLLIS DILLER

Maintaining a sense of humor about cooking is very important. In the past, women (and often men) were expected to be able to cook and serve an appetizing meal. Now it seems that the skills run more toward being able to make skillful choices at the carryout, choosing items that won't "blend" when heated up in the microwave.

Seriously, though, eating is serious business and we do not need to be serious about it. So many people have so much strange energy about food, and so many people grew up in families where the favorite place for stress release was around the dinner table that we have become very confused about eating in general.

Just a few reminders:

1. *Eating is fun.*
2. *Food tastes good.*
3. *Food can be a form of adventure.*
4. *Food can be healthy and delicious.*
5. *Plastic is not food.*
6. *Save serious conversations for a time when you do not have a table between you for protection.*

Meals can be regrouping and rebalancing times. Are yours?

BLAME

Fair play is primarily not blaming others for anything that is wrong with us.

ERIC HOFFER

In a world of psychological "reasons" of why this or that happened and why we are the way we are, it is anything but easy not to blame others (*any* others!) for what is wrong with us.

We can spend so many years believing that we never had a chance because of poverty, divorced parents, poor education, overindulgent parents, or unfortunate life circumstances that we continually end up blaming someone—*anyone*—for our lot in life. We may hold some deep-seated belief that if we can prove we have been unfairly treated, then we are absolved from dealing with others fairly.

Each thought or word of blame we think or utter reduces the quantum of "fairness" residing within us. If we are not careful, we may draw on our fair-play pool so much that we have little reserves left.

Don't despair! Fair-play reservoirs are easily replenished. All we have to do is quit blaming others for what is wrong with us and quit feeding our thinking along these lines. It's amazing how modeling fair play elicits a like response in others.

Make a note to raise a mental red flag when you start blaming someone else for anything.

FEAR OF CHILDREN

Hedda was queasily phobic of children and, by extension, of short people in general. They were too condensed, like undiluted cans of soup—too intensely human and, therefore, too intensely not to be trusted. The mistakes in the basic ingredients—the stupidity, the cruelty—were overpoweringly present.

REBECCA GOLDSTEIN

It's not easy for most adults to admit that down deep we are afraid of children. Modern psychology has planted the seed that children are creatures to be feared, and that seed has fallen on fertile ground. We have been encouraged to focus upon children as the repository of our unfocused and unnamed fears.

What in the world are children doing, and what goes on in those minds? If we do or say anything, we can harm them. If we do not follow all the parenting experts, we will do something wrong. Are they trying to manipulate us? Are they really sick or malingering? *Who and what are these little people anyway?*

Whew! We seem to have forgotten that we were once children. Were we so dangerous? Perhaps we were unknown to ourselves and chances are we can remember a time when we knew exactly who we were.

Relax. Let the "experts" believe their fears. Kids like to relate to real people, not papier-mâché characters.

See if you can relax and be yourself with a child. It's great practice.

INNOVATIONS

After I started living my life more as a process, I decided to take a cot to the office so I could take a nap every afternoon. I needed it. My boss didn't mind.

REINHOLD

For Reinhold and the publisher for whom he worked, his taking a cot to the office was a revolutionary act. He worked in a company with a strong work (and overwork!) ethic. Yet over the years, he had proven himself a good producer and a steady, reliable worker. After the cot, his production was as good or better than before. His self-caring act sent out shock waves in the company, prompting others to look for ways to help them work more sanely and creatively. They, too, began to move in new directions.

Reinhold did not drag his cot to his office in order to be an innovator. He did so because as he gradually became more aware of himself and his needs and was willing to try to meet those needs in ways that were not harmful to anyone (or his work!), he decided that the cot was a good solution.

In a quiet, subtle way, he became an innovator in his workplace.

Good innovations start with need.

Tune in to yourself. What would make your workplace more humane for you?

ILLUSIONS

I always think that I can take time to rest when the work is done and the work is never done.

PETRA

Illusions are very tricky. They creep in when we are not looking, they keep themselves hidden until we are vulnerable and unaware, and then they spring into action with the fierceness of a caged lion.

Most of us can't remember when we started harboring illusions. Usually they come into our minds through family, church, schools, and all forms of the media with theories espoused by current psychology. As illusions grow in our minds, we begin to feel at home with them and freely participate in the process of building our own.

Take for example, the illusion that there will be a time when the work is done. There is *never* a time when the work is done. Life and work are processes constructed in such a way that neither is really done until life is over. That's the way it is. We can complete little pieces of work and there will always be more work. Our issue is to learn to take care of ourselves in the process of doing our work.

Build an "illusion sweeper" and start to clear the illusions out of your mind.

DIGNITY

Throughout all her bitter years of slavery (my mother) managed to preserve a queenlike dignity.

MARY McLEOD BETHUNE

What an ancient relic of a concept—dignity. We rarely hear much about dignity in this age of *casual* and *grunge*. Yet, when we see true dignity, we often feel awe and appreciation.

True dignity is not trying to create an impression or impress others. True dignity is a process of inner balancing that allows us to move through life on life's terms while respecting our own terms.

Too often when we think of dignity we think of the stiff rigidity of Victorian women and want nothing to do with that. Thank goodness! Dignity has nothing to do with rigidity.

Dignity is the ability to fine-tune to our internal gyroscope of balance regardless of what the world throws at us and to respond with clarity and compassion for ourselves and others. Dignity is the ability to let down our hair and play with the best of them while maintaining our selfhood. Dignity is being ourselves and responding to the situation.

Sit down and think of some people you believe have dignity. You might want to check out yourself.

BEING A HOLLOW BONE

[W]hen we become hollow bones there is no limit to what the Higher Powers can do in and through us in spiritual things.

FRANK FOOLS CROW

Of all the things my grandfather, Frank Fools Crow (Eagle Bear), taught me, the importance of being a hollow bone was the most profound and, I believe, the most valuable.

Fools Crow was the most important healer and spiritual leader I have known thus far in my lifetime. Yet, he would be the last person to claim either, for he was very clear that everything he did came from Higher Powers. He was a powerful man, and his power came from his knowing that he was a hollow bone and from his practicing that he was a hollow bone. Because of his knowledge that he was a hollow bone for the Great Mystery, he lived ninety-eight years of healing spiritual service. His life was filled with gentle humility. He had everything he needed and was loved and admired by many throughout the world.

Living our lives as hollow bones means that our egos and personalities step out of the way and we open up our lives to be guided by powers greater than ourselves. When we do this, a peace and balance like no other descends upon us.

Sit down and look back over your life. See if you can see times when you thought everything was perfect and you wanted to keep it that way forever. You failed, of course. Your life moved on. See if you can recognize how much more you have learned and how much richer your life has been than if you had successfully kept it static. Then contemplate the possibility of being a hollow bone.

EXPANDING OURSELVES

What is the color of wind?

ZEN KOAN

The purpose of a Zen koan is to teach, to stretch, to expand, to puzzle our minds into new perceptions.

What is the color of wind? What is the smell of a piece of music?

So often, we limit the possibilities of our experience by staying in the ruts we have deceptively decorated to look like living rooms, while the world around us offers us myriad possibilities for living that we do not even allow our senses to perceive.

We are so extraordinary as human beings! We have more possibilities in every moment than we can imagine. And we can live those possibilities even if we have not let ourselves perceive them.

When we recognize how creative we are and how vital and alive the world around us is, we open up more possibilities.

Today, try sitting in a familiar place and opening your senses and your being to the unusual and heretofore unknown present around you.

SILENCE

To be able to listen to the silence is to be able to hear the infinite.
ANNE WILSON SCHAEF

Silence is one of our most valuable gifts. And, so many of us have not known being listened to, that when we speak of the value of silence the concept falls on deaf ears.

Perhaps we need to learn that we have a voice in order to appreciate the true value of silence.

Too often, in order to have a voice, we have learned to debate, argue, be assertive, and con people. We have learned to speak over others, to start preparing what we will say next to "win." Yet, after all these skills have been learned and practiced, we feel strangely empty inside. Although the very skills we have been taught may work in certain situations, we need to ask ourselves whether they are effective generally. Do we feel good about ourselves and others when we use them? Are we talking to hear ourselves talk, to avoid the silence, or to prove how much we know? If it is because of any of these, it is better to be silent.

Once we have learned to speak what is important to us, we will find more beauty in silence.

Silence is almost a lost experience in today's society. See if you can develop a way of listening to what is being said in such a way that nothing is required of you. Conserve your power.

EUPHEMISMS

I know uh secret code. I ain' crazy, I got uh 'motional disorder; I ain' got fits, I got uh convulsive disorder; an' I ain' ugly, I plain; an' I ain' black, I dusky; an' my children ain' bastards, they—they love-flowers!

JOANNE GREENBERG

What, you may ask, is a meditation on euphemisms doing in a book on living in balance for people who do too much? I asked myself the same thing.

Euphemisms was close to *euthanasia* in the book of quotations I thumbed through, and I discovered that I like both words. Aren't they fun? Eu-phem-isms, eu-than-na-sia (or is it na-s-i-a?). What fun! Don't you love words?

In an old Cinderella movie, *The Glass Slipper*, the fairy godmother was a very believable, normal-looking, old round woman who loved words. Windowsill *(winnnn-do-silll)*, pickle relish—words are *fun*. They can be so much more fun when we just play with them. Foool-ish, fool-ish, full-ish.

Isn't it full to be foolish once in a while and just play around with something?

Euphemisms are funny anyway. They're like lying—like trying to say something without saying it. Now isn't that silly?

Try being foolish and silly. Do something meaningless—and enjoy it while you're doing it.

PERSEVERANCE

Perseverance is not a long race; it is many short races one after another.

WALTER ELLIOTT

People who do too much have trouble with perseverance. We like to hurry up, get something finished, and get on to something else—something *new*.

People who do too much are not good plodders. We enjoy the excitement and the adrenaline of the rush and the push

Unfortunately, when we rush and push, our sense of balance suffers greatly. We are so focused on one motion—forward—that our sense of balance in all spheres, at all levels, and in all directions becomes distorted. We may be going around in circles and it is usually in one place or circles hopping wildly from one place to another. We lose ourselves in the process.

Two approaches can help us:

1. *Knowing that we can take only one step at a time and focusing on that step, taking it as completely and fully as we can.*

2. *Breaking up the task in small pieces that are doable and building on the tasks that are already done.*

When you are faced with a task of long duration, try breaking it up into doable segments, taking one step at a time.

MONEY

There are a handful of people whom money won't spoil, and we all count ourselves among them.

MIGNON MCLAUGHLIN

Ah, money! What illusions! What fantasies! What dreams we have about money! It is amazing that we are willing to put so much time and energy into something that isn't even real.

Money is something that we have made up, seeing it as real is a cherished cultural illusion. When we stand back and look at money from a larger perspective, we really are a little silly about it, aren't we?

Yet, one of the strangest and most peculiar characteristics I have discovered about money is that it is completely devoid of spirituality. Dealing with it over long periods of time depletes our spirituality.

We have developed a myth about money. The myth goes like this: money is neither good nor bad, it's what you do with it that counts. This is a favorite myth developed to cover this and other nonspiritual things.

I propose that dealing with money depletes our life energy. How do we feel after a siege of paying bills? How do we feel when we are trying to straighten out a mixed-up credit card statement? How do we feel after doing our taxes or meeting with retirement consultants? My experience is that I feel spiritually depleted. Money is a great imbalancer, whether we have a little or a lot.

> Try "sandwiching" your money tasks with something spiritual—a reading, a prayer, a meditation, a walk in nature—before and after. See if you experience a difference in the way you feel.

HEALTH—BODIES

Health is not simply the absence of sickness.
HANNAH GREEN

Health and balance are not static. Balancing our bodies means paying attention to all the phases of our bodies and of our lives. What is balanced at one phase of our lives might not be balanced at another.

Neither balance nor our bodies are static. Our bodies are constantly moving, changing, living, dying, and rebuilding. What is balanced for one person may not be balanced for another. There is really no static image of a healthy body. As much as we would like to believe the contrary, there is no such thing as an agreed-upon balanced body. Our bodies are a reflection of the process of the self that inhabits them.

Our bodies are like our lives. They are not an "it" that can be fixed up perfectly and will remain that way. Our bodies and our health are processes. If we try to get them fixed up and hope they will stay that way, we are participating in one of life's favorite illusions. Our bodies are not machines; they are processes. We get along better when we treat them as processes.

Try to start thinking of your body as a process, not as an "it." See if this changes the way you relate to it. We can work with our bodies. They are not our enemies.

SELF-ESTEEM—TRUTH

The brother that gets me is going to get one hell of a fabulous woman.

ARETHA FRANKLIN

Right! There's nothing like the truth. All too often we get the mistaken idea that expressing the truth involves only expressing the negatives about ourselves. If it is the truth, it's got to hurt—or so we think.

When we express the truth about the good things about ourselves, we are told that we are bragging or that we are conceited. Now where is the balance (or truth) in *that*?

Every one of us is a full, talented, whole, creative human being. Every one of us is a fabulous person with potentials that have barely been tapped.

Whoever gets us for partners or for friends is a lucky person. We may have some rough edges and they are just obvious signs of our potential for growth.

Spend the day recognizing that you are indeed a fabulous person (along with whatever else you want to think about yourself today).

SELF-CENTEREDNESS

There is no such thing as balance. How I long for that sense of repose after a good day's work. Does anyone have it?

NAOMI THORNTON

How utterly human! Just because we don't know how to do something and have not found a way to work it out, we come to the conclusion that it doesn't exist! Black Elk said that "the center of the universe is everywhere." He didn't say, "*I* am the center of the universe." The center of the universe may be within me, as it is everywhere, *and* I am not it!

Self-centeredness is so limiting and so destructive. Self-centeredness is not taking care of oneself, as some believe. It is the process of being out of touch with oneself while focusing completely on the "I." Self-centeredness is like a black hole that leaves no room for the self or the other. The state of self-centeredness is so powerful that it expands to fill in whatever space is there. People who live around self-centeredness often become self-centered themselves because they reach a state where they begin to feel that they have to grab something for themselves. In this way self-centeredness is contagious. The worst thing about self-centeredness is that when we are immersed in it, we don't know it—and we haven't a clue how to get out of it.

If you suspect self-centeredness, stop, take stock, talk to a friend, and do something purely for someone else.

DIFFERENCES

Differences challenge assumptions.
ANNE WILSON SCHAEF

Succumbing to fear of differences is a very good way to stay static.

When we have to deal with someone who is very different from ourselves, we tend to retreat to distancing strategies. We see differences and immediately pull back into ourselves. We secretly and silently affirm who and what we are and our way of doing things, and we judge the other person for being different.

Why are we so afraid? Do we have to remake everyone else in our own image to feel comfortable with them? Our natural human tendency in new and unknown situations is to try to reach into our "knowns," and define the situation from that perspective.

Yet, there are other ways of dealing with our fear of the unknown. Challenging our assumptions may be just what we need. We can see and feel the differences, acknowledge our fear to ourselves (and even to others), relax after that acknowledgment, open ourselves to stretching and/or discarding our assumptions, and prepare for something different—even unknown.

Do most of the people in your life look and act like you? If so, is this uniformity a celestial imbalancer? Do you want to look at the way you have constructed your life with respect to differences? This could be a cutting edge for you.

MAKING ASSUMPTIONS

Assumptions are dangerous things.
AGATHA CHRISTIE

Assumptions can be very dangerous, especially when we act on them without checking them out. "I thought you were finished so I cleared the table and cleaned off your plate." "I thought you weren't interested so I went ahead without you." "I thought you were going to leave this relationship anyway so I let you go." I have heard it said that assumptions are premeditated resentments, and I believe it's true. "I just assumed you wanted to go so I said yes." "I assumed your going to bed with me was some kind of commitment." "Since you didn't get back to me right away, I assumed you thought I wasn't the right person for the job."

How easy it would be to check out our assumptions before acting upon them! A simple phone call, a visit, a fax, or an email would be enough.

Wars (personal and international) have been started over un-checked-out assumptions. We need to be very careful about assuming anything about anything.

Check out your assumptions. Try to take one day and be aware of your making assumptions and/or acting on them. Look at the results. This assumption-making may be something you need to consider.

RELATIONSHIPS

Relationships cannot be controlled. We can participate in their happening.

ANNE

Sometimes, we confuse relationships with magic.

We wish for relationships that are intimate, loving, open, gentle, and supportive. Our first choice would be to find just the right person and magically enter into the perfect relationship, then have it continue flawlessly so that we can get on with the other, more important things in our lives. We hope that we can fix up our relationships once and for all, just like we would like to do with our houses, and have them stay that way forever. Although most of us would say that we do not believe in magic, we want our wishes and desires to come about magically, especially in our relationships.

How silly we are! Intimacy takes time. Intimacy is a process, not an event. Intimacy is something in which we participate, not something we are given.

Schedule a once-a-week check-in with the most intimate person in your life. In between, take a look at what you have done to cause or contribute to tension and be ready to own that behavior.

SETTING LIMITS

Work expands to fill the time available for its completion.
C. NORTHCOTE PARKINSON

I am of the firm conviction that the papers on my desk reproduce at night. When I leave them, they are sorted neatly and stacked to be attacked later. They don't seem daunting and overwhelming. Then, in the fresh light of day, they seem to have expanded in an attempt to demand more of me and fill my life as fully as they can. Papers and work have a way of doing this—completely on their own. It's their nature.

Once I recognized this phenomenon, I realized that I had to take full responsibility for my papers and my work. Since I had discovered the secret nature of their being—to expand themselves exponentially—it became my responsibility to set boundaries to curb their essential nature, which was not always good for my life, my relationships, or my health.

When I know that I have a potentially endlessly growing phenomenon on my hands, I can do what I need to do to see that I do not let this natural phenomenon overrun my life.

When I leave my desk, I warn the papers to be chaste—no reproducing!—and I clearly tell my work that I have set limits and will not fall prey to its essential nature. It's like training a puppy.

Speak to your papers or the dishes in the sink and let them know that you set the limits here. Check in occasionally to see that they are following orders.

PASSION

I began to bring the passion I had for basketball to the [General Motors] meetings.

CYNTHIA "COOP" COOPER

All too often when we think of serenity and balance, we confuse these states with a passionless life.

To people who have lived on the edge, pushed the envelope, wrestled with life, and lived on drama, crisis, and adrenaline, balance and boring seem to go together.

Surprisingly, perhaps to some anyway, living in balance is not possible without passion. We may have confused passion and adrenaline. Passion is the laser-like focusing of our creative life force, infusing it with enthusiasm, filling it with energy, seasoning it with love, and living it with aplomb.

We do not create passion. It wells up within us like an overflowing spring when we allow it. Let's not confuse passion with overdoing or with workaholism. Workaholism devours while passion enlivens. Our passion does not require us to be destructive to ourselves for its sake.

Passion is the true vehicle for aliveness.

Look at your life. Where are your passions? Have you lost some of your passion? Is it there in a different form than it was in your youth? What can you do to support your passions? Commit to letting yourself be a passionate person.

THE RIGHT TOOL FOR THE JOB

Work is no longer a place.
JARMA ALLILA, CHAIRMAN AND CEO OF NOKIA

We used to think in terms of our workplace as a location where we did our work, whether that was at home or in the office. Much of that has changed with the advent of the electronic age. We have much more opportunity for freedom of place, and much more opportunity for chaos, clutter, distractions, and losing things.

The busy mom may have not only an at-home place that's her work corner or office. She may also find herself "doing business" while she waits to pick up kids in the carpool or while standing in line at the checkout counter.

The business executive may do as much on the commute as she does in the office. The teacher may make calls to parents while he sits waiting for a family member at the dentist. Times have changed!

Cell phones, faxes, and emails have given us a different sense of place. We need to see what gear we need for a mobile office. Throwing a cell phone and notes into an old purse may do more harm than good. Your beloved old briefcases may benefit from a few folders with overflies.

See what accessories you can find that can support the style of your life right now. These are always good investments. I like portfolios—the kind with lots of pockets—that fit into my briefcases.

CIRCUMSTANCES

Circumstances don't make a person, they reveal him or her.
RICHARD CARLSON

What we do with the circumstances of our lives reveals who we are. We are not created and molded by the circumstances of our birth and our subsequent life. They may influence us and they do not make us. The most important element is who we are and how we respond. There is no need to belabor here the many stories of similar people with almost identical advantages and how they end up with very different outcomes for their lives.

It is our responsibility to create what is possible for us with what we have. What we do with what is offered to us is our opportunity to reveal who we are and who we can become. The opportunity and the responsibility are ours.

When we begin to get some perspective on our lives, we can see the result of some of the choices we have made. This offers us the opportunity to grow from our mistakes *and* our successes. It is the perspective that adds balance to our lives.

Sit back and see what you have done with the circumstances you were given. Are there changes you want to make now?

CHALLENGES TO BALANCE

To him every form of life that he encountered was both an admired and good neighbor, even those classified as "exceedingly dangerous and deadly."

J. ALLEN BOONE

What would happen to our sense of balance if we saw every form of life we encounter as an "admired and good neighbor"? Take cockroaches, for example. That's a tough one, isn't it? There is some speculation that if the world were overcome by radiation, the cockroaches might be the only ones to survive. I have known people who seemed to live easily with cockroaches as well as those who swore that they talked with the cockroaches and asked them to leave and they did. I have not found it easy to see cockroaches as my neighbor and teacher, though at times I have managed. Yet, what changes would there be in me if I could see them as part of a whole creation of which I am only a part?

I have found this process of seeing mosquitoes as family somewhat easier, and lately most mosquitoes have little interest in biting me.

I have little opportunity to be around creatures classified as "exceedingly dangerous and deadly" (except people, of course, and I do see the Creator's hand there).

Most of all, from a meditation like this, I see how far I have to go and how much I have to learn. That's always a good thing.

Where do you need to push your boundaries with respect to all creation? Is it in the way you see a neighbor, an ex-spouse, or a bug? There's always some opportunity to move toward balancing our attitudes.

ANIMALS—PETS

Animals do not betray; they do not exploit; they do not oppress; they do not enslave; they do not sin. They have their being, and their being is honest, and who can say this of man?

TAYLOR CALDWELL

How lucky we are to have or to have had pets in our lives! It's not just that they have been there to love and be with us (though many of them have done just that!). What if we shift our perspective a little bit and open ourselves to the possibility that our pets have chosen us because we needed them at a particular point in our lives? Perhaps our pets have volunteered to be our teachers because our lives were too rigid or too narrow or too lonely and we needed something that was not easy to come by.

As children, many of us learn about unconditional love from our pets. They are always there, and they seem to love us no matter what. We learn about acceptance. They accept and forgive and are frequently called upon to do this with us. On the other hand, we often find it easier to accept and forgive our pets than we would another human being.

Pets teach us about the better aspects of being human and let us practice learning our humanity. They add balance to our lives. What more could we ask?

Do something good and/or important for an animal every week.

JUDGMENTS— JUDGMENTALISM— COMPASSION

Make no judgments where you have no compassion.
ANNE MCCAFFREY

One of the ways we throw ourselves out of balance is by being confused about the difference between making a judgment and being judgmental. The two are vastly different, and recognizing the difference can be very important to our peaceful living.

We have to make judgments all the time in order to participate in life. Do we want the salad, the soup, or the sandwich—or two or three? Do we want the ATV, the four-door sedan, the station wagon, or the convertible? Life is full of everyday judgments we need to make for life to proceed smoothly.

Judgmentalism is making judgments with a high level of negative energy attached. Not only do we not want the salad; the salad is *bad*. It's not just that we prefer the four-door sedan; the others are *no good*. It's not that we choose not to be around a certain person; we have to make that person bad and then try to convince others that our opinion is right. Judgmentalism involves making heavily weighted negative judgments without the wisdom and perspective of compassion. Judgmentalism will throw us and those around us out of balance.

Distinguish between judgments and judgmentalism for yourself. Learn to nip judgmentalism in the bud.

WATER

In all the years when I did not know what to believe in and therefore preferred to leave all beliefs alone, whenever I came to a place where living water welled up, blessedly cold and sweet and pure, from the earth's dark bosom, I felt that after all it must be wrong not to believe in anything.

SIGRID UNDSET

The sound of running water has the ability to calm all our demons and return us to a level of serenity as nothing else can do.

Water has so many voices. There is the peaceful burbling of a brook as it tumbles over rocks and moves to its home, the sea. There is the rush of rapids as they gather speed in their headlong thrust of movement. There is the steady call of the waterfall, masking all "unnecessary" noise. And, there is the glorious thrashing of rain as it torrents and peppers our windows.

Regardless of its form, water lulls us back to ourselves, inviting us to return to hidden inner rhythms that get lost in rushing.

If you don't have your own stream or waterfall, it's very easy to get a little personal "fountain" that will share the sound of water with you for years to come. You might want to check one out.

LOSS

Losing is the price we pay for living. It is also the source of much of our growth and gain.

JUDITH VIORST

Learning to live in balance requires that we learn to deal with loss and separation. Although we experience many gains in living, often it is the losses that we try to ignore and avoid. We have a tendency to want to hold on to everything we have ever had—people, places, things, ideas . . . even characters in novels or movies.

Learning to deal graciously with loss is one of the more exciting challenges in life, and the process of this learning allows us to move deeper into the full meaning of life.

Favorite clothes, family, friends, jobs, everything that exists materially—all these are always under the threat of loss. How much easier our lives become when we recognize and accept this process: pets die, friends move away, houses are sold.

When we face loss, we need to take the time to feel and process our grief. Grief is not only normal; it is part of the healing process of loss. I knew a woman who always grieved the end of a good book, as the characters would no longer be actively in her life. She taught me a lot.

Remember, grief takes time. It does not fit itself into anyone else's schedule. We need to honor grief and give grief the time it needs, and then learn and grow from our loss.

How do you deal with loss? See if you have old griefs that you have not honored, then write about them or talk them over with someone.

COMPASSION

If you want others to be happy, practice compassion. If you want to be happy, practice compassion.

DALAI LAMA

For so many of us, compassion is an abstract concept. We believe that it is probably a good thing, and we know that saints and other such beings are noted for it. Yet, we find it difficult to bring compassion down to our very human, everyday level.

In German, the word for compassion is *mitfühlen*—literally, "to feel with." This is not to feel for, to do for, to take care of, or to fix. Compassion is "feeling with." It's that simple. How much more balanced and meaningful our lives would be if we could "feel with" those around us.

One of the ways to learn to feel with is to get to know others beyond a superficial level. When we experience another's life the way he or she experiences it, our world expands and we begin to develop the ability to feel with. We develop compassion.

All too often we avoid feeling with because we are afraid of the pain and the sorrow we will encounter. We forget that we are robbing ourselves of the joy and creativity that are also there. No life is just one thing or one way. We are all multidimensional.

Open yourself to "feeling with" others. You'll not regret it. If necessary, put yourself in some situations that you have previously avoided in order to do this.

PRAYER

What we usually pray to God is not that His will be done, but that He approve ours.

HELGA BERGOLD GROSS

Let's face it: we human beings are a funny lot. We want help, no doubt about that (and we *need* it, too), and we usually want help (when we can admit at all that we need it) when we want it and in a form that *we* predetermine, and in a way that we recognize it as help. When we are finally willing to ask for help, the preconditions are so staggering that one can imagine even God having difficulty interpreting all the fine print. We want to be in control of things about which we know very little and for which we can't possibly have the perspective to know all the variables and options.

We're not too eager to ride around with a blind person driving the car, and yet we are willing to have a deaf, blind, uninformed person (us!) controlling our lives. Now you have to admit—that's funny.

Prayer seems complex to those who are unfamiliar with it or think too much about it. However, it is very simple for those who have walked in its path steadfastly. Prayer is very simply this: "Thy will be done" (or "the ball's in your court and don't expect me to return it with much finesse").

Try praying (while flat on your back before you start and after you end the day, if possible) "Thy will be done" and see what happens. Don't think too much.

GRIEF AND JOY

It is difficult to define grief as joy. Each is finite. Each will fade.
JIM BISHOP

Grief and joy are both processes. Both will come, and both will go. Both have the potential to flow through our lives, flushing us clean and leaving us open for new life and new experiences. Both are good.

It's good that we can grieve. The ability to grieve is an extraordinary gift. Grief allows us to celebrate our intimacies and acknowledge our losses. Whether we are grieving for the loss of a loved one or for the ending of a good malt, grief is a wonderful, appropriate response. Grief cleanses us, affirms our ability to love, and prepares us to move on with life.

Joy is much the same. It affirms both our humanity and our divinity. Joy connects us with all that is while reminding us that we have the ability to soar beyond the stars. Joy is true aliveness unfettered by thought.

The difference between grief and joy is what we do with them. Grief we push away. Joy we try to hold on to. When we refuse our grief, it stays. When we try to control our joy, it leaves. That's the way these processes are.

Take a look at the way you have treated grief and joy in your life.

NATURE AS WISDOM

Nature never says one thing and wisdom another.

JUVENAL

In our busy, responsible, and intense lives, one of the first things we filter out is our time in nature. Our bodies are surrounded by asphalt, steel, and concrete, and our lives become crowded by things and activities. Even if we love nature, we find ourselves spending less and less quality time there, perhaps simply popping in for a quick fix of sanity on weekends and holidays. Interestingly, many people as they grow older seem to find time to be in nature, realizing the importance of that time.

Many years ago I was told by an old Cherokee Medicine Man, "When you are ready, come to me and I will teach you. I will take you into nature; you can learn everything you need to know there." I'm sure that he didn't mean Outward Bound or a ropes course. He just meant nature.

Nature has a wisdom that transcends time and space, a wisdom that is expressed in a powerful quietude of simplicity. In nature we have the extraordinary possibility to delve into a shared wisdom deep within ourselves.

Bring nature to you in plants and flowers, and take as much time as you can to go into nature. A walk in nature at least three times a week is a good start.

SHAPING AND BEING SHAPED BY OUR SPACE

We shape our dwellings, and afterwards our dwellings shape us.
WINSTON CHURCHILL

I have always been amused by the concept of completely designing and deciding upon a building project or remodeling, and then holding on to the belief that it will go exactly as planned. Builders and planning commissioners have yet to recognize the reality that in the *process* of building, perspectives and realities change.

A home should *feel* good, and often we do not know how something *feels* until we feel it. A design for a bathroom may fit all the most up-to-date architectural and code standards and look great on paper. Yet, as it begins to emerge in reality, it may not "work" for us.

Whether we build a space or move into one, once we're there we need to participate in the "shaping" process with our dwellings. We need to let ourselves feel the energies of the rooms to see what works. We need to try out various possibilities and see what feels good for us and what feels good with the space. If we insist on imposing our perceptions and preconceived notions on a room, it will be cold and uninviting.

It is the interacting of these mutual shapings that makes a house, an apartment, or an office a home. Intellectual ideas and concepts never quite do the trick.

Check out your living space and your working space. Have you participated in shaping and being shaped by them?

DOUBLE-SPEAK

It's no exaggeration to say the undecideds could go one way or the other.

GEORGE BUSH

There is something about this statement that hits us right where we live. What a comfort to know that the undecideds can go one way or the other. What is the definition of an undecided, anyway?

In modern times, our lives can easily become unbalanced by listening to doublespeak, and even more so by doing it.

Double-speak is giving the impression that you are saying something—even something vitally important—when you are not saying anything at all. Double-speak is most effectively used in situations where we don't want to be held responsible for anything that comes out of our mouths and believe that we can accomplish this. Double-speak is a form of escaping while standing in one place. Many have spent years developing this form of communication, believing it to be a skill. People who are *really* good at this form of communication can do double-speak without saying anything at all.

The problem with double-speak is that the speaker and the listener both are required to abandon themselves to tolerate it. Double-speak is not a form of communication. It is a form of assassination—of the soul.

Check yourself and those around you for double-speak. See how it feels and make choices.

LISTENING

Wisdom is the reward you get for a lifetime of listening when you'd have preferred to talk.

DOUG LARSON

Listening may be one of the most important activities we can choose to participate in in our entire lives.

Listening—really good listening—involves a great deal more than our ears. To listen, we need to empty ourselves for a while. We need to adjourn the committee in our heads and invite its members to take an extended vacation. In order to listen fully, we have to be able to dismiss idle head chatter, criticism, and judgmentalism. Otherwise, our heads are far too crowded to have room for anything new.

We have to open our hearts as well. The absolute very best listening is done with our hearts, not our heads. We have to be willing to let the words enter our beings, where they can be tenderly sifted and sorted so that we are available to know the various levels of their true meaning.

Then, we have to be willing to open our beings so that the deep crevices of our ancient, connected minds can caress that which goes beyond the frail utterance of words.

Listening is a highly complex and intimate process.

Practice opening your mind, heart, and being. You'll hear more than you imagined possible.

PARENTING

Our children need to know that we are not perfect, and it's better if they hear it from us.

ANNE WILSON SCHAEF

We parents are some of the best cons in the world. Regardless of how enlightened we are, we have great reluctance for our children to see our imperfections. It's not that we are completely unwilling for them to see *all* of our imperfections. Heavens no! We are quite willing for them to see those that we are *comfortable* with their seeing. It's the others that give us problems. Also, we are usually quite creative in our reasons for not admitting to our wrongdoing. "*They* couldn't deal with it." "Knowing would damage our relationship." "We made a mistake and won't do it again, so why disturb them with it?"

Several years ago, my son taught me a lot about this. He had gone into a teenage withdrawal, and I went crazy thinking about what terrible things might be going on. So . . . I snooped. I admit it. I snooped. I convinced myself that I was justified, and, true, some of my fears were realized, so I could focus on him for a while. And deep down I was raging within myself. I had put myself in a position I didn't like, and I hated it. When I finally quit focusing on him, I realized that I needed to tell him what I had done, apologize, and risk losing his trust. When he saw the pain I was in for this breach of my values, and the pain and fear I felt at risking our relationship (which I valued like life itself), he was more able to feel safe to admit his issues.

Modeling is the most important thing we can do for our children.

Take a hard look at what you are modeling for your children.

SELF-CENTEREDNESS

*I see how my self-centeredness keeps me from knowing that
I am loved.*

SANDY

How silly we are sometimes! We are so busy wanting people to love us—believing that we can control *who* will love us, *when*, *in what way*, and *under what conditions*; being afraid that people *will* love us, resulting in a huge list of demands that we don't want to meet; being so sure that we really down deep are not lovable and that when people get to know us they will walk away—that we don't take the time to stop to see that we have people in our lives who already *do* love us.

When we are self-centered, down deep we believe that if we did not create it (whatever *it* is!) or make it happen, it simply does not and will not exist. We are so busy trying to get our needs met that we fail to see the possibility of more abundance than we could imagine (or control!) all around us.

We can't see the world around us because we spend so much time being in our own way.

Try another approach. Get up and do something for someone else.

GOD DOES FOR US WHAT WE CANNOT DO FOR OURSELVES

I had to let my office go and I kept on working and ignoring that fact. Then when I had no choice, I looked for a bigger house where I could have my home and my office. I found one and then when I had to move out of my office, the house deal fell through. All my office stuff is now stacked in my garage.

PETER

We often hear the phrase "God does for us what we cannot do for ourselves."

As brilliant as we are, we never will quite have the whole picture. What may have seemed our most brilliant decisions or solutions at the moment would have turned out to be disasters if we had been able to carry them out. At times like this, some celestial hand seems to intervene to stop us from digging ourselves in any deeper. We may not like it at the time, but, with a little more perspective, we can see that our best-laid plans would have been disastrous.

Take Peter, for instance. He is a retired person who has not fully retired from his workaholism. When he is functioning with clarity, he is a well-known artist in his spare time. If he had moved his business office into his house, he would never have had a moment's peace. He would have been working all the time. Lucky for him, something intervened.

Look back on your life and remember those moments when your lovely plans did not go the way you thought you wanted and yet life turned out better.

NOURISHING DREAMS AND VISIONS

Champions aren't made in gyms. Champions are made from something they have deep inside them—a desire, a dream, a vision.

MUHAMMAD ALI

We have become confused about what champions are and what makes a champion. The corporate world has propagated the illusion that the champions—those who get ahead—are the ones who work the hardest and the longest, never taking any time for themselves or their families. The illusion is that to be successful, one must be driven and ruthless, putting work above everything else. Unfortunately, this notion has permeated our work lives and resulted in a generation of burnt-out workaholics. And yet productivity and workaholism have little in common.

To be productive, to be a champion, one must tap into that deep wellspring inside that nurtures dreams, visions, and desires. To have desire without vision is like growing a plant without water. A plant needs water to flourish, and the process of absorbing the water takes time. The water has to be put into the soil, then it seeps down to the roots. The roots slowly take in the water, at the same time absorbing minerals and nutrients from the soil. Then the slow process of this water and nourishment moving up to the full plant begins. Nourishing dreams and visions takes time. Yet it is dreams and visions that make us true champions.

What are your dreams and visions?

UNIQUENESS

The reason Wakan Tanka does not make two birds . . . or two human beings exactly alike is because each is placed here . . . to be an independent individual to rely on himself.

OKUTE

Each of us is a unique individual. Not only are we unique to begin with, the experience we have in living can never be duplicated by anyone else. We are a unique combination of the DNA of our ancestors and the experiences we have created and lived each day of our lives.

Because of our uniqueness, each and every one of us is responsible for the balance that is necessary to make the whole.

The universe is like a big puzzle in which every part of creation has a place. When we fail to take our place, there is a hole in the universe. As we take our place, we become part of the whole and realize that while we are unique, we are also part of a whole that is much greater than ourselves. With these two realizations—of our uniqueness and of our being an integral part of a greater process—we achieve a sense of inner balance.

Today, express your uniqueness and your connectedness in what you do. Come up with a new idea or a new way of doing something. Then, reflect on it and see how it builds on gifts you have learned from others.

WAITING

Sitting quietly, doing nothing, spring comes, and the grass grows by itself.

ZEN SAYING

One of the ways to find balance in our lives is to realize that we don't have to do it (whatever "it" is) all by ourselves, and we do not have to do it at once.

Many tasks and issues in our lives will take care of themselves if we will but let them. The "impossible" task that *had* to be accomplished immediately looks very different tomorrow or next week. Often, I have found that when others are pushing something as *urgent*, setting a definite time limit, my best response is just to slow down. For one thing, I do not always make my best decisions under those circumstances (and, I must say, I have observed that others don't either!). My decision to take my time is not always popular with those around me, and they have to deal with their feelings about that. Taking my time may mean that I miss a deadline or an opportunity and, if I do, I have learned to trust the outcome, whatever it is, and to live with it. Almost always, new information arises to support my having waited.

One of the hardest decisions in this modern world is to do nothing, and doing nothing is often a big improvement over frantic activity.

Practice "when in doubt, don't" for a few days and see what happens.

ANGER

Anger is a symptom, a way of cloaking and expressing feelings too awful to experience directly—hurt, bitterness, grief, and, most of all, fear.

JOAN RIVERS

Anger and all of our other emotions are gifts that we have been given to open doors into deeper and deeper levels of ourselves. Emotions and feelings are the pathways beyond the rational, thinking mind that lead us to levels of spirituality not readily accessed.

Anger is not a "negative emotion." Anger just *is.* It's what we do with our anger that's important. If we randomly dump it on others, we are not only quite likely to get a backlash, we are probably going to feel bad about ourselves.

When we cease to be afraid of our anger, when we cease to have the need to justify it, and when we cease to spew it, we have the possibility to see it as the door that it is and to let it take us down that dim path that leads to the light of spirituality and wisdom.

The next time you feel angry, don't spew it. Welcome your anger and let it take you through and beyond feelings that may need to be healed to places of light.

CRITICISM—POSITIVISM

They never raised a statue to a critic.

MARTHA GRAHAM

Criticism and cynicism are national diseases. And, this doesn't mean that people who do too much have to overburden themselves with them.

Although criticism and analysis are still seen as sophisticated and scientific, we *do* have other choices. For example we can vaccinate ourselves against their contagion with positivism. We can silence our inner critic. The choice is ours. Being critical rarely results in improvement; it usually results in anger and distrust. We can catch ourselves in the act of being critical and take another tack. We can ignore our negative thoughts rather than feed them on grains of criticism. We can accept flaws and what needs to be changed while shifting our focus to positives and goodness.

Being critical can become a habit, and habits are easier to make than break. Being positive can become a habit too. We can be grateful for what we have, for who another person is, for what we have received, and for what we have learned.

When we replace the negative with the positive, subtle and significant shifts begin to occur, like huge fissures in a glacier.

Try noticing your inner critic, silencing it, and replacing it with something positive and see what happens.

LETTING GO, HOLDING ON

If I can let you go as trees let go / . . . Lose what I lose to keep what I can keep, / The strong root still alive under the snow, / Love will endure—if I can let you go.

MAY SARTON

What beautiful words! What an important concept!

We so often distort ourselves and throw ourselves completely out of balance by trying to hold on to something or someone that needs to go or is already gone—a job, a thing, a person, a life.

Expecting that *anything* will last forever is one of the more dangerous things we do to ourselves. How much of our time and energy is spent trying to hold on?

We don't just try to hold on to people. We try to hold on to things. We need to let ourselves remember that things wear out, break, and get lost. That's just the way it is. Jobs wear out, break, and get lost. Relationships wear out, break, and get lost.

We can shift our perspective. We can be grateful for the experience and time we had and let go of the person or thing. Celebrate the pleasure. Celebrate the experience. Celebrate the sharing. And then accept the loss and let go.

In the process, we may shift our perceptions and our expectations.

See if there are persons, experiences, objects, jobs, or relationships you are holding on to that are finished. Are you ready to let go?

MISTAKES

If I had my life to live over, I'd dare to make more mistakes next time.

NADINE STAIR

Careful, careful—don't make mistakes. Careful, careful—if we *make* a mistake, we *are* a mistake. Maybe if we overdo, overwork, do as much as we can, people won't notice the mistakes (or, if they notice, they will forgive them because we are doing so much).

Watch it! Control it! Keep it safe!

Ironically, trying not to make a mistake is probably the biggest mistake we can make. Mistakes aren't bad. They just *are*. We are not mistakes ourselves; we just make them.

I know this may come to a shock to some and mistakes can be fun. I have noticed that when I feel really grounded and in balance, I almost welcome mistakes. I most certainly get excited about them. Seen through balanced eyes, they are our opportunity to learn, to grow, to expand.

Being cautious, on the other hand, can be stifling!

When you find yourself being fearful and overly cautious, indulge in a mistake. Take risks. Try the untried and learn from it. Whee!

RESENTMENTS

I discovered something important last night: I create my own resentments. I was lying there awake and tired because my dog is sick and keeps waking up at night. As I lay there, I started thinking about things that were perfectly all right before I started thinking, and then I began to build resentments.

CONNIE

What a powerful discovery: we create our own resentments—and out of nothing!

Have you ever noticed that sometimes someone does something and it doesn't bug you at all? Then, a few moments (or months) later, that or some other person will do the same thing and you hate it? The situation is the same. We are the ones who have changed. When we keep the focus where it belongs, on ourselves, we can see that our reactions are just that—*our* reactions. When we see that our resentments are just that—*our* resentments—we can see the possibility of relief. If we built them, we can change them. If we built them, we can dismantle them. It's all so simple if we don't try to muck things up by making others responsible for our resentments.

This is not in any way meant to imply that others don't do awful things. Of course they do. *They'll* have to deal with that. Our resentments hurt *us*, and *we'll* have to deal with that.

HALT. Don't get too Hungry, Angry, Lonely, or Tired. These are fertile grounds for resentments. When you start building a resentment edifice, check out HALT and start dismantling. Otherwise, the edifice will fall on you.

PRACTICAL REGROUNDING

The grass is spring green, tall and full of newborn life, waving in the breeze. I can smell its fragrance, and this purely physical sensation helps me let go of other thoughts and centers me here.

OLGA KHARITIDI

Sometimes the physical and an awareness of it is what we need to center ourselves.

The airplane wobbles and we grab for the armrests. We feel our lives spinning out of control and we just have to plop ourselves down on the ground. We feel off-kilter and we go clean the stove or sweep the floor. We feel rushed to a point of suicide and we hug our child.

There is something about the physical world around us that can help ground us when nothing else seems real. Our thoughts rush frantically to "get a grip," and the taste of tea is what we need.

So often it is the practical physical activity of doing something that provides the mystical solution for irrational situations.

Feel overwhelmed? Go brush your teeth, sweep a floor, fix a sandwich (and savor it)—do something practical to reground yourself.

FAULTS

The fault no child ever loses is the one he was most punished for.
MIGNON MCLAUGHLIN

It's not our faults that throw us off balance. It's how we think about them.

Many of us have become tenaciously attached to our faults. They have become part of our identity. There was so much emphasis put on them and attention paid to them when we were children that we would feel lost without them. In fact, some of our faults were basic survival mechanisms that allowed us to grow up in dysfunctional families. Conning, being "good boys and girls," stubbornness, isolation, dishonesty, fear, and self-centeredness may have been our best friends and essential for our survival. How could we continue to exist without them?

Good question. They have helped us exist. Now are they keeping us from living? Is it time to let them go and move on? The very thought may strike panic in our bones.

Like everything else, our faults can be our teachers. Just because we see faults in ourselves doesn't mean we can't also be great. In fact, our very recognition of our faults may significantly contribute to our greatness.

What are the faults that bug you the most about yourself?
(If you have trouble coming up with any, you may want to
ask family and friends!) List them. Take a good, hard look at
them. See what is your attachment to each. See whether you
are ready to let it go.

ACCEPTANCE

You kinda have to work with what you got and accept what you get.
HURRICANE FLOYD SURVIVOR

These words from a woman standing in the mud next to her wrecked home and business sounded pretty profound to me.

How much easier our lives would be if we could "work with what we got and accept what we get"!

Working with what we have is not always easy. First we have to see what we have. I worked for a man once who was the best administrator I have ever known. He ran the department in an easy, casual way, encouraging each of us to be creative, productive professionals. He himself was a high producer, yet he never put any pressure on his employees. He respected their gifts and uniqueness and was good at what he did.

Unfortunately, he didn't *value* his excellent skills! He wanted to be a theorizer and creative thinker. He was always restless and dissatisfied.

He was good at accepting what he would get in employees, and he was not good at valuing and honoring what *he* had.

When we use what we have and accept what we get, life flows.

Take a look at your attitude toward working with what you have and accepting what you get.

ANGER

No one, Dora thought, could get through the violent tedium of young, daily married life, without becoming angry, so that the very way a husband ate a meal could become a matter for thought-murder.

POLLY DEVLIN

Anger is such a powerful, wonderful emotion. It's a pity that we waste it on those we love when we could do so much more with it!

Actually, anger probably has little or nothing to do with those near and dear to us. The coward in us has taken the easy way out, dumping it on those closest to us instead of gearing up our courage and facing off with it ourselves.

Anger often simmers up in us as a warning, a signal that we need to pay attention to our internal life. If we don't, anger will wreak havoc on our external lives.

Anger is a warning light, to go to into ourselves. It is a glowing signal breaking through the shroud of darkness we have fashioned in our lives. Anger offers an opportunity to learn something about ourselves, to use the blade of our wrath to plow the field of our learning rather than to strike down those we love. Anger is our friend when we honor it and don't dump it on others.

The next time you feel angry, don't dump your anger on others. Go off by yourself, sink into it—rage if you must—and let yourself be open to whatever lies beneath your anger. You may be surprised—pleasantly—by what comes into consciousness.

DEALING WITH CRITICISM AND SELF-DOUBT

One thing I never do is doubt myself. . . . I don't beat myself up like that. I have confidence in myself and my ability, and then whatever happens is the Lord's will.

CYNTHIA "COOP" COOPER

So few of us have really mastered the difference between accepting and checking out criticism and doubting ourselves. Doubting or not doubting ourselves is much deeper than accepting criticism. In fact, it is only when we have a deep, abiding relationship with ourselves—that trusts that we can take in, check out, handle, and clearly accept or reject criticism—that we come not to doubt ourselves. When we are defensive, we clearly don't trust ourselves enough to examine criticism, sorting it out, keeping what is useful, and tossing the rest. It helps a great deal to know that we have some sort of Higher Power we can ultimately turn the issue over to after we have done our part.

As we go through this process, we learn to trust ourselves. Beating ourselves up is only self-centered self-indulgence. Who needs it? When we learn to have confidence in ourselves and our abilities, we can leave the outcome to the powers that be.

What do you do with criticism? When you get into a cycle of self-doubt, try stepping back, being open to any truth in the criticism, checking it out, taking what is useful, and pitching the rest, knowing that you've done what you can. Avoid brooding.

HOPE

There are no hopeless situations; there are only men who have grown hopeless about them.

CLARE BOOTHE LUCE

One of the things that silently falls by the wayside when our busy lives get stretched too thin is hope. Hope is never limited to the unreal. Hope is that process within ourselves that stretches us beyond the ordinary, beyond the possible to the impossible, while at the same time rendering what seemed impossible possible. Hope feeds our soul and our being. It is that immeasurable source of power that comes from beyond ourselves and is not controlled by us.

Depriving ourselves of hope confines us to a world grown devoid of color and surprises. We no longer see the flowers and the rainbows that are there.

Hope is not expensive to have. It is very costly to be without.

Hope is one of the inalienable gifts we have as human beings. It can never be squandered or overused.

Whenever you feel desperate or hopeless, recognize and accept that feeling. Let yourself know how that feeling is there to open the possibility for hope to reenter your life.

ACCEPTING IMPERFECTIONS

*That is why humility—the knowledge of our own imperfections—
is so important, and that is why spirituality goes on and on and on,
a never-ending adventure of coming to know ourselves, seeing ourselves clearly, learning to be at home with ourselves.*

ERNEST KURTZ AND KATHERINE KETCHAM

There is a difference between seeing our imperfections as bad
and seeing them as a given of reality that offers us an opportunity.

When we get caught in the myth of perfectionism, we see
our faults as glaring and horrible reminders that we are not as
we should be, that we have failed and are indeed *ourselves* failures. This point of view doesn't leave much room for humility,
forgiveness, love, acceptance, or growth. In short, this view is
pretty self-destructive. Our imperfections are not the problem;
our attitude toward them is. This negative attitude toward the
reality of imperfection is fertile ground for self-hate and nega-
tivism toward others.

When we accept our imperfections, we can with humility
participate in that "never-ending journey of coming to know
ourselves." To know ourselves, we need to be willing to drop
the veils of illusion that we have wound about ourselves, give
up our denial, and come to accept ourselves as we are. The irony
is that as we accept ourselves as we are, we become freer to
change and grow and become *better* than we are.

Funny how it works.

*Take a little time each day to list what you see as your imper-
fections. Be aware of your attitude toward them. Practice
acceptance.*

SELF-UNDERSTANDING

I do not want the peace which passeth understanding, I want the understanding which bringeth peace.

HELEN KELLER

The greatest journey we will ever take is the journey into ourselves, for we are a microcosm of all that is. We can learn (and we need to learn) from all that is around us. Self-understanding is what will bring us the peace of balance.

Self-understanding rarely comes from thinking or analyzing ourselves. Self-understanding is not self-absorbed navel-gazing. Self-understanding is soul awareness. It comes with allowing that knowledge that is within us to emerge.

So many brilliant and gifted people squander their gifts because they lack the humility of self-understanding. When we think we know it all, we miss the point. When we think we know everything about ourselves, we show our ignorance and our arrogance. The wonder of human beings is that we are constructed in such a way that we can spend our entire lives exploring our inner universe and its connection to the universe as a whole and still barely scratch the surface.

We are a wonder for us to behold.

Never stop learning about yourself or you will be an uninformed fool who has no peace. Self-understanding is a process that is never completed. We fool ourselves when we think we have had enough.

WORRY

I have been through some terrible things in my life, some of which actually happened.

MARK TWAIN

Frantic—worry—rush. Frantic—worry—rush. We have set up our lives as if we were running on a hamster wheel enclosed in the cage of our own frantic rush and worry. As with the little hamster, so often it seems as if we run but never get anywhere. Our running keeps us so busy and distracted that progress eludes us.

Worry is one of those "hamster wheels" of our lives, offering us the opportunity to live through terrible things that never happen. When we stop to catch our breath, we might ask ourselves, "Why *pre*-worry?" "Why live through something that hasn't happened and may never happen?" Do we actually believe that worry practice will make us better prepared?

Remember, everything has a beginning and an ending. We only need to deal with situations in our lives as they are happening, not before.

Today's disaster may tomorrow or next week be seen as one of life's gifts. All we have to do is deal with what is in front of us.

When you start to worry, stop to see if you are in the past or in the future. If either, focus on the present and see what you need to do—right now.

MENTORS—HUMILITY

Some women find mentoring valuable not only in helping them move ahead but in keeping them from dropping out.

SUSAN CAMINITI

"I have to do this on my own." "If I were good enough, I wouldn't need help."

Where in the world do we get these ideas? Even John Wayne needed a complete cast of characters—a director, a producer, and hundreds of "little people"—to make him look like the self-made hero.

All of us have had mentors. Admit it! We have! Generations of people have backed us up to get us where we are now. None of us is completely self-made. We may have had the courage and intelligence to grasp the moment, and yet that moment would not have been there if others had not gone before, clearing the way for us and giving us seen and unseen support.

We would not be here if it were not for the DNA and genes of our ancestors. That's a fact. Remembering this helps put our life in perspective.

We would not be able to do what we have done without the inventors, teachers, and creative geniuses who developed the building blocks on which our work is based.

We would not have learned without parents and teachers, good and bad, who helped us figure out who we want to be and who we don't want to be.

We didn't get here by ourselves.

Today would be a good day to stop to recognize the role that others have played in our lives, our heritage, and the support we have been given. It's good humility training.

LISTENING TO OURSELVES

The only listening that counts is that of the talker who alternately absorbs and expresses ideas.

AGNES REPPLIER

When we want someone to listen to us, we want to be heard—no doubt about it. And, often, the real issue is that we want the opportunity to put our words, ideas, and feelings out into the world so that *we* can hear and see them.

Some of us are very auditory (and all of us are auditory to a certain extent). We often become slightly unbalanced in our visually dominated world.

We need to *hear* what we are feeling to make it real enough to deal with. We need to *hear* what we think in order to roll our thoughts around and build on our ideas. We need to *hear* our observations so *we* can weigh them in perceiving reality. We need to listen to ourselves, and one of the best ways to do that is to talk to someone who is a good listener.

Find someone to talk to who will support your listening to yourself.

DIVERSITY

Diversity is the most basic principle of creation. No two snowflakes, blades of grass, or people are alike.

LYNN MARIA LAITALA

Diversity is the mother of balance.

It's odd how we can nurture the illusion that balance and sameness are identical. Sameness feeds our illusion of control. Diversity, on the other hand, offers us the creativity of balancing-unbalancing-rebalancing. Balance is an ongoing process. It is not static. We don't achieve balance and then ignore it, going on to better things. Balance is an ongoing process in which we can participate. The diversity in our lives and around us offers us many of our best options for balancing and rebalancing.

As human beings, we push and push and push for sameness, not really seeing that this contributes to our feelings of imbalance. We want to be around people who are similar to us. We want our culture to cover the globe. When we travel, we want to stay in accommodations that are "familiar" to us. We want our children to marry someone like us.

We may like the idea of diversity, and yet we want the practicality of sameness!

Stop to assess the ways in which you invite diversity into your life. How could you include more diversity? Are you open to explore diversity? Read some books or articles by people unlike yourself. Go to some places you would not usually visit. Even try diversifying your food. See what happens.

PRAYER

Certain thoughts are prayers. There are moments when, whatever the attitude of the body, the soul is on its knees.

VICTOR HUGO

Sometimes, it seems as if the role of organized religion has been to remove prayer from the everyday and make it a special "holy." For some unknown reason, many of us have become convinced that we have to be taught to pray. Not only do we have to be taught, there is a right way and a wrong way, and we had better not do it the wrong way. Though rarely stated, there is a not-so-subtle message that God, the great teacher in the sky, is standing up there marking a scorecard on each life, with everything we do counting as a test. "This one gets an A in prayer. This one gets an F and will have to repeat this life in the same school. This one is definitely prayer-challenged and needs remedial work." Did I pass? *Did I pass?*

Good heavens! No wonder we shudder at even trying!

Frankly, we need to quit listening to the "experts." If God created all of creation and we're included in that (though some would like to be superior to the rest of creation), then we have a direct connection. We don't have to be perfect; we only have to participate . . . then something gets through.

What is your attitude toward prayer? Has your concept of prayer been diminished by what you have been told? How about getting back to the basics?

MIRACLES

Who does not believe in miracles in this holy land is not realistic.
DAVID BEN-GURION

Ben Gurion uttered these words about Israel as it became a state.

To dispute the existence of miracles is to dispute the existence of the processes of life. Can anyone who has marveled at the tiny hands of a newborn baby not believe in miracles? Every sprout that comes forth from a seed is a proclamation of miracles.

Miracles occur not only outside of us; we know them internally every day. Is it not a miracle that our inner beings in their infinite wisdom store memories in our minds and bodies for us to work through when we have reached the level of awareness, strength, and maturity to deal with them? Often, when things happen to us, we are not ready or able to deal with them and so we "forget." And, they wait there, seemingly dormant, until we are ready to move through the feelings and experiences to "heal" that particular incident. This healing process, inherent in all of us, is a miracle.

Our bodies and our minds—our beings—are all miracles.

The next time you take your morning pee, realize what a miracle it is that your kidneys function.

BOASTING

Boast is always a cry of despair except in the young, when it is a cry of hope.

BERNARD BERENSON

Isn't it fun when we see something that has always been decidedly negative given a positive slant?

Take boasting, for instance. Most of us have been trained to believe that boasting is not good and that we don't look good when we boast. Yet, here's a man who says that in the young it is a cry of hope. How good for the young to have a cry of hope!

Perhaps boasting has gotten a bad rap. Perhaps even the label *boasting* has been applied incorrectly. For example, there is a general rule of thumb that says we are not supposed to say we are good at something (even if we know we are very good at it) in order to avoid the horrible sin of boasting. Now, that puts us in a senseless bind. It seems that convention says it is infinitely better to lie than it is to "boast" the truth. What nonsense!

Because we have confused boasting with telling the truth, we have thrown ourselves and those around us out of balance. Boasting requires a certain amount of conceit and dishonesty. Telling the truth about our assets requires humility and honesty. We don't need to lie about the truth.

Be truthful about yourself. Try, just once, saying "I do that well" when you do.

RESPECT FOR LIVING THINGS

To us, our house was not unsentient matter—it had a heart, and a soul, and eyes to see us with; and approvals and solicitudes and deep sympathies; it was of us, and we were in its confidence, and lived in its grace and in the peace of its benediction. We never came home from an absence that its face did not lighten up and speak out its eloquent welcome and we could not enter it unmoved.

MARK TWAIN

What a shift we make toward balance when we begin to realize the sentience in the quiet energies around us!

Several years ago a group of us bought an old hot-springs hotel in Montana as a place where individuals could come for healing, a place that was not controlled by professionals. The initial healing that needed to happen was with the building itself. The magnificent old structure had been abused, neglected, and ignored. It had leaks in the roof and in the exterior walls. The historic roof was red and patching it would mean matching colors. Then one member of the group said, "Why are we talking about patching the roof? This old lady needs a new red hat." Suddenly we knew our answer. We needed to convince the old building of our intentions and respect. After that decision, as I drove from the back of the building around to the front, I was aware that the hotel was glowing and smiling. We then had its cooperation.

Remember that houses, cars, and clothes all come from living materials endowed with energy. Our lives become simpler when we treat them with love and respect.

Look around you. What things in your life have cared for you? Recognize and affirm this caring. Return it if you can.

WATER

My old friend, water, my good companion, my beloved mother and father: I am its most natural offspring.

DORIS GRUMBACH

Throughout the ages water has been considered a great healer. We begin our lives in the waters of our mother's womb. We are born of water, a large percentage of our bodies is water, and water helps us digest and carry what we need throughout our bodies. We need water physically, psychologically, and spiritually.

We can have many healing relationships with water. One of them is bathing. Over the last few years I have had the marvelous opportunity of visiting various spas in Europe where the warm mineral water pours freely from the earth. At one of these, there is a loosely structured process of about eighteen steps of different kinds of bathing. The first step is a required eight- to twelve-minute shower followed by a warm sauna (sweating fifteen minutes), a hot sauna (five minutes), another shower, a soap brush scrub, a shower, steam room, a shower, a soaking shower, and so on, ending with a total dousing of lotion and a twenty-minute blanket-enfolded sleep. I have never felt so *clean!* And I realize that my efficient showers at home just do not have the same effect.

Bathing, showering, soaking—we need to let water be an important part of our lives.

Treat yourself to a long session with water.

GARDENING

Perennials are the ones that grow like weeds, biennials are the ones that die this year instead of next, and hardy annuals are the ones that never come up at all.

KATHARINE WHITEHORN

Now here is a woman who knows about gardening!

I have sat for hours listening to friends and acquaintances talk about the peaceful, rejuvenating aspects of gardening. They extol the rapture of digging in the earth with their hands (their fingernails must have fallen off years ago; perhaps those are fake things at the ends of their fingers, to be removed before their next foray into their dirty gardens!).

I have listened carefully as others (who seem to know what they are doing) discuss in detail which plants are compatible and how annuals, biennials, and perennials should be placed in a garden. I don't know what happens to me in these conversations. My mind retreats to the same dark, blank place it goes to during discussions of theories about world economics.

I have asked for help and found that most of the people who respond to my cry are "theoretical gardeners," people who would rather talk about gardening than do it.

I like flowers and fresh herbs. My solution has been to buy flowers and hire a gardener. As a result, I have strong, pretty fingernails.

When you like the product but not the process, see if someone else can do the process.

We don't have to enjoy everything. Filter out one supposed-to-be-good-for-you thing that you don't enjoy.

LISTENING

No man was ever wise by chance.

SENECA

There seems to be a one-to-one positive correlation between wisdom, listening, and humility. The wisest people I have ever known have also been the most humble and skilled listeners I have ever known. Somehow listening, wisdom, and humility seem to form an unstoppable tripod of basics for good living.

As I have observed good listeners and thus learned to be a better listener myself (I'm Irish, and we Irish love to talk!), I have had time to see some commonalities in good listeners that seem important.

First of all, good listeners have the ability to listen to themselves. They are not selfish or self-centered in their self-listening. They are simply attentive. They are attentive to the small stirrings within themselves that allow them to know themselves and to be in tune with themselves.

Second, they listen to their God, their Higher Power, their Creator, or the Universal Wisdom that sustains and informs us all.

Third, they listen lovingly to others, finding something of importance in everything that is said.

And last, they listen to nature, knowing that the utterings of the world around them are older than any of us and need to be heeded if we are to live in balance and harmony.

Practice the four basics of listening spelled out above and see if this kind of listening makes positive changes in your life.

CHILDREN

Perhaps parents would enjoy their children more if they stopped to realize that the film of childhood can never be run through for a second showing.

EVELYN NOWN

Perhaps God gives us children not so much to perpetuate the human race; God gives us children to give us companions who will make every possible effort to help us remember to be fully present and to live in the present.

Children are the ultimate reminders that life is nothing more than a process, and that as we participate in it, it changes. Children are willing to take on people who have started to become static, to busy themselves with unimportant things, and to lose contact with the world around them.

We are given children to help us remember to *live* our lives, not just rush through them. Contrary to the belief that children bring imbalance into our otherwise ordered lives, children shake us out of the narcolepsy of detached, rote-performance living. Children simply won't put up with detachment.

Watch a bug with a child or watch a child watching a bug.

WORKING FUN

Working is more fun than sitting around worrying about money.
PETE

The other day, a group of us were sitting around talking about the various jobs we'd had when we were younger and how much fun we'd had with them.

We started out with working-during-college stories. A couple of us had worked as nurse's aides in hospitals. We recounted the late-night shift on a wing for old nuns and the satisfaction we'd felt in learning to distinguish the sound of each individual bell as the old women summoned help in the middle of the night.

We shared a flying-nun story, when two of us had a wild and noisy time with a huge floor-waxer that took possession of us for a brief moment. Our shrieks of laughter disturbed the head nun. We tried to get ourselves under control, as we could hear the approach of the stiff, white, starched habit descending upon us from down the hall. With absolutely no innocence at all, when reprimanded, we said that we did not know how to use the floor-waxer (we had already had the experience of being flung around by it!). She took the bait, saying that it couldn't possibly be *that* hard. To our delight, she grabbed the handles ordering us to plug in the cord. The result: a flying nun! By this time, patients and staff had gathered, we were told to pull the plug and forget the incident . . . as obviously I have!

In the course of that recent conversation, we remembered what fun we had had in various jobs, from waitressing to emptying bedpans, and we were reminded how much fun working can be.

Let yourself reminisce about the fun you have had with jobs in times past.

LOST PERSPECTIVES

When I was working on the tour, I found myself really getting into my workaholism. I got completely crazy and found the only thing that helped was to call a group of my friends together to talk and help me get back my perspective.

ULRIKE

How easy it is to lose our perspective when we are under stress. Just when we most need support and help, we often decide to focus doggedly on the task at hand. We look neither left nor right. We take on the characteristics of a tyrant, expecting everything in our environment to modify itself around what we are doing. Suddenly, we and our work become the center of the universe, and we are often truly surprised when others don't see "reality" the same way we do.

Just when we need other input the most, we isolate, pull into ourselves, and develop a laserlike focus on what *has* to be done.

This is when we need to stop, call friends together, and get a reality check. Reality checks are great for getting back perspectives.

The next time you get deeply task-oriented take a reality-check break with friends, family, or co-workers.

CHANGE

I thought I could change the world. It took me a hundred years to figure out I can't change the world. I can only change Bessie. And honey, that ain't easy either.

BESSIE DELANY

There's the problem! Unfortunately, some of us just may not live long enough to learn this lesson!

It is so easy to see what is wrong "out there" and expend all our energies trying to change people, places, and things (and keeping *terribly* busy doing it!), never taking the time to see how *we* need to change to make our lives and the lives of those around us better.

After we have expended our energies on the impossible, we have the opportunity in the quiet of exhaustion to see what is possible. Often what is possible in even the worst of circumstances is changing and shifting our attitude and perspective. When we do that, doors begin to open that were not even visible to us before.

We human beings are so dear. We often take forever to see the obvious, and we often get quite bloody in the process.

Take a problem situation you have been trying to resolve and instead of obsessing and trying to control it, see if you can truly shift your attitude or perception of it and see what happens.

RUNAWAY MINDS

We don't have to say or think what we don't wish to. We have a choice in those things, and we have to realize that and practice using that choice.

ROLLING THUNDER

How can we achieve balance if we see ourselves as victims of our own thinking? All too often we give ourselves permission to let our thoughts run rampant. Say we call a friend who is busy and doesn't want to talk right then. Our thinking shifts into self-centeredness, and we decide that she really doesn't want to talk with us at all and that we are not going to put ourselves in the position of being humiliated again, so we don't call back. Our thoughts drive us crazy. Then, months later, we run into her on the street and she greets us with great warmth, throwing her arms around us and telling us how glad she is to see us. She also shares that she has been ill, as have members of her family, so her plate has been overflowing. Our thinking has tricked us! Suddenly we realize that not only have we missed her, we have missed the opportunity to have contact with her and maybe even to have been of help to her.

We are not at the mercy of what we think or what comes out of our mouths. We may have crazy thoughts at times and it is up to us whether we indulge in them or not. Our balance is in our hands, in conjunction with the Great Mystery, of course.

Practice not indulging in a runaway mind. Set up a red-flag system for yourself so that you can identify times when you begin obsessing about something.

EMPTINESS—RELATIONSHIPS

We shape clay into a pot, but it is the emptiness inside that holds whatever we want.

TAO TE CHING

Modern society has developed a cultural need to be filled up. We want more food, more alcohol, more drugs; we have come to believe that we need more money, more things, more sex, more power—more, more, more.

We are so afraid of any emptiness that we feel inside that any awareness of this void sends us scurrying to fill it up . . . with anything—just fill it up.

Yet, there is no way to experience balance in our lives with constant and continued fullness.

We need to learn to be aware of and to value our places of emptiness.

For example, so many people when they leave a relationship either already have another one warming up in the bullpen or they immediately scurry around to "attach" to someone, frequently making a bad choice.

It is normal and good to feel an emptiness and loss when a relationship ends. Taking the time to experience the void, the loneliness, and the loss will more than pay off in the years to come.

When we accept the balancing of emptiness in our lives, we begin to have a better knowing of the *Is.*

Each day has many losses. Take the time to know and experience them.

HANDING IT OVER

Pase lo que pase la vida sigue su curso.
Regardless of what happens, life will continue.

MEXICAN PROVERB

Sometimes, it's the simple little things that bring us back into balance. The complex concepts and the flowery phrases may be intriguing and beautiful, and, when our lives seem off-kilter and out of balance, it is so often the simple things that hit the mark.

When there are no words, as at the death of a child, I have heard the above words uttered and they healed with their simplicity. *No matter what, life goes on.*

When we feel as if we are at the bottom, and we no longer have the illusion that we can *make* our lives go on, we are strangely comforted to know that we are not in charge. Life will go on with or without us.

For those of us who like to run things (and who doesn't, deep down?), there is a deep relief in knowing that we really don't, and really *can't*, take the helm. We just don't have the qualifications for the job! Not having to run everything can give us the option of doing what we can, resting, or—whatever.

Let the proverb "Regardless of what happens, life will continue" sink into your being. Remember that there is always a new day ahead.

CONTROL

You take people as far as they will go, not as far as you would like them to go.

JEANNETTE RANKIN

I had an experience recently that helped me learn something about control. I went to a group in which I participate, one in which decisions are supposed to be reached by consensus. There is one person in the group who not only never seems to hear what others want to do, she actually seems only to hear what she wants to do and *believes* that others have said the same. I always react inside when she does this, but I can let it go fairly quickly (sometimes better than others, I must admit). I see her as very controlling.

After the group, she and I chatted; we talked about marriage, living with other people, and so forth, and she said, "Don't complain about spouses." She went on to tell me about a friend of hers who lives alone but doesn't feel complete without a man and desperately wants to be married.

"How awful," I said, having worked through that particular cultural brainwashing (as I saw it) years ago.

"Not necessarily," she said. "That's where she is, and that's what she's working through right now."

Bingo!

Often it takes someone who has what we see as a whopper of a negative characteristic (in this case, control) for us to see it in ourselves.

We can indeed only take people as far as *they* will go. Our illusion of control is creative.

Check out your illusion of control. What are some of the more subtle and creative ways you have developed to try to control others?

ADVENTURE

Adventure is worthwhile in itself.

AMELIA EARHART

And she was certainly an adventurer! Not all of us will be Amelia Earharts and we can all be adventurers.

Perhaps the most exciting adventure that any of us can have is the adventure of an ordinary day.

Life is made up of ordinary days made extraordinary by what we do with them. We have that power.

We truly see in life what we want to see in it. Every day we have the possibility to see the amazing all around us. There are the faces on the bus, in the crowd, or at the store. When we really look at them, they become extraordinary.

There is the holiness in common things too. The water pouring out of the faucet, the clean feeling we have when brushing our teeth, or the sweet explosion in our mouth when we bite into a piece of fruit—all these are holy experiences.

We also have the potential to scatter joy and compliments around like fairy dust everywhere we go. What could be more adventuresome?

See what adventures you can have on this day. Don't forget your fairy-dust scatterer.

WHAT'S IMPORTANT

We have the task of building two things while we are in our physical lives. Our first task is to construct the physical reality in which we live. The second task is the creation of ourselves—of that very self that lives within this outer reality.

Both sides require attention. Keeping the balance between them is a very sacred and demanding art. As soon as we forget one task, the other can capture us and make us its slave forever.

OLGA KHARITIDI

There are many ways to look at what's important in life. What's essential, however, is to let ourselves *see* what's important. No matter how we conceptualize what's important for ourselves, the concept of balance is always in there someplace. Kharitidi was told of two realities, both of which involved many factors.

We need to live in our physical world. That's our reality. So we need to find, build, and develop a physical reality in which we can live, thrive, grow, and learn. Making our own peculiar, comfortable nest is essential for us. Yet, this process of creating our physical reality will never be satisfying for us if it is at the expense of our second reality: the creation of ourselves.

The creation of ourselves demands that we go deep within, facing our demons, exploring our depths, and soaring with our infiniteness.

We need the balance.

Just looking at your life from the perspective of the construction of the physical reality and the creation of yourself, do you have balance?

STUBBORNNESS

In the face of an obstacle which is impossible to overcome, stubbornness is stupid.

SIMONE DE BEAUVOIR

Ah, stubbornness! It's one of those wonderful little friends we have developed that may have been our tools for survival at an earlier age and are now killing us. Oh, how we hate to give them up, don't we? Remember, we never really have to give anything up until we're ready, and stubborn people have a very difficult time becoming ready. Also, when we are so busy, we have the perfect excuse not to have the time to take a look at some of our "old friend" traits that are killing us the fastest.

Usually, we can get some great physical clues about our stubbornness. Our jaws clench, our hands curl tightly, our lips get thin, our head muscles squeeze, our backs straighten and stiffen, our shoulders hunch, and our butts tighten. Are we having fun yet? Ah, yes, I forgot the squinting and the narrowing of the eyes. Even our ears seem to close. Stubbornness is hard on the body as well as on relationships.

We have our agenda, and we're not going to change it. Most important, if we look, we see ourselves becoming persons we don't want to be, persons we don't even like! Is it worth it? We have other options.

No one ever expired from letting go of stubbornness.

Sit down and write out a few of your most stubborn positions. Are you willing to move off dead center on them? Check it out. You and your friends and family will be glad you did.

FINANCES

I believe that one's basic financial attitudes are—like a tendency toward fat knees—probably formed in utero, or, at the very least, in cribbo.

PEG BRACKEN

Being balanced with respect to finances requires high levels of emotional, mathematical, economic, and managerial skill. There are very few people who don't feel overwhelmed by finances. So relax. Don't think you're so unique (that's dangerous thinking—there is an identified syndrome called "terminal uniqueness"!). Dealing with finances isn't just making and spending money. It's not even just avoiding becoming obsessed or emotionally enmeshed with money (though these can be problems too).

Dealing with our finances in a balanced way means that we back off, get a bigger perspective, remembering that creative finances may resemble a shell game—so *observe*, and don't play.

Being balanced with our finances in this day and age may mean talking to a whole array of experts, most of whom *may* have some piece of the puzzle and many of whom have not even realized there *is* a three-dimensional puzzle. Accountants, tax consultants, retirement consultants, actuaries, lawyers, Social Security people, investors—the list is so long that this process needs to be started at an early age.

Then, when you have gathered tons of opinions and some information, the final step is to relax and do what makes sense to you.

What do you need to do to bring your finances into balance with the rest of your life?

WONDER

If I had influence with the good fairy who is supposed to preside over the christening of all children I should ask that her gift to each child in the world be a sense of wonder so indestructible that it would last throughout life, as an unfailing antidote against the boredom and disenchantments of later years, the sterile preoccupation with things that are artificial, the alienation from the sources of our strength.

RACHEL CARSON

How precious is our sense of wonder!

Wonder is one of the great balancers of human experience. Our sense of wonder protects us from forgetting that reality is relative and that perceived realities are influenced by our beliefs. Our sense of wonder gives us the foundation to stick with our deep knowing of our reality even when it isn't seen or shared by some around us. Wonder helps us remember that we can become so embroiled in what seems to be the practical that we lose sight of the important. Wonder connects with the unseen forces that create and guide our lives. It is the door to beyond that we need to return to here.

We can't afford to get in a position of wondering where our wonder went.

Do a "wonder assessment." Have you seen yours lately? If not, get help. Animals, new babies, budding nature, and adults who have incorporated all the ages they have thus far been are helpful guides.

BEING CLEVER

Para un largo hay otro más largo.
For every clever person, there is a person more clever.

MEXICAN PROVERB

Sometimes we people who do too much just need to be put in our place. When we get off balance, we vacillate from one end or the other of one of our favorite dualisms—being worthless versus being the greatest thing in the world. Of course, whenever we are caught on this dualism, no matter which end we favor we are always out of balance.

It's a certain relief to know that there will always be people more "worthless" than we are and others who are more "clever." This knowledge relieves us of the responsibility of being the "most," freeing us up to deal with our reality. There will always be those who know more than we do about something. This doesn't mean we know nothing, nor does it mean we have to know *everything.* We can know what we know. We can be as clever as we are. The possibility of balance is inside of us—not external to us.

Whenever you are feeling like a "hot shot," remember the above proverb. Whenever you are feeling useless, remember the other end of the dualism.

FAMILIES

The great gift of family life is to be intimately acquainted with people you might never even introduce yourself to, had life not done it for you.

KENDALL HAILEY

Have you ever stopped to look around your family and had the frightening notion, "Who *are* these people?" Well, they're the people you are with in this life who offer you the most intimate playground possible to work out the game of life. They may not be the family members you would have chosen. And, they are the ones you have. When you realize that the issue is not focusing on them and what's wrong with them or on who you would rather be, and that the issue is that this family is the rich grist for your learning mill, your perceptions might change.

What can you learn from each one? What are qualities that you like? What are qualities that you would rather not be around? Which of both do you share with them (be honest now!)?

When you have started to "see" them, is there room for compassion in you?

They are not the cause of your present pains. They are the triggers for dealing with it.

Families are blessings we can choose to bless in return.

Step back and get a clearer perspective of your family. Honor whatever feelings come up and be open to learning from them.

THINKING

Sit down, shut up, and give your brain a rest.

ANONYMOUS AA SPONSOR

There's nothing like a direct order to help us get back in balance!

One of our greatest "imbalances" is our thinking. Our minds are great—don't get me wrong. And, our thinking can get us in more trouble than we sometimes believe. The truth is that we can almost never think our way out of a problem. Typically, the more we try to solve it with our thinking, the deeper we get into it.

Our brains have a secret magnifying glass that turns even the most microscopic issue into an earth-shattering problem. Our thinking has a power of magnification that would be envied by the users of the world's greatest telescopes. Usually, when our mouths chew on something it becomes smaller. Yet, when our brains chew on something, it grows bigger and bigger. By the time our brains quit chewing on an issue, it has become insurmountable to our psyches *and* our spirits.

When we start getting into this spiral of thinking, the best thing we can do is sit down, shut up, and give our brains a rest.

Listening to others is a great antidote to our thinking.

Spend a day listening to others without adding your important piece. You'll be amazed with the results.

OFF BALANCE

When I am into my workaholism, I can't even take time to talk with my partner or a friend on the phone. I always rush through the conversation and cut it short.

ROLAND

One of the devastating side effects of getting too busy and doing too much is that our brains become confused and we lose track of what is important.

Our brains are amazing. They can find ways to rationalize and justify almost anything we want to do. If we want to work ourselves to death, our brains can give us a reason that sounds perfectly logical and rational—it just doesn't make any sense. If we want to get so busy that we don't have any time to talk to our partners or our friends, our brains can make that behavior okay in the moment, rationalizing that as soon as this spurt of work is over, we will again take more time for them.

It's not really that we *want* to neglect spouses and friends. We have just moved off balance and need to rebalance ourselves.

Call a friend today and take time to be present to the conversation.

THE OBVIOUS

Her greatest skill was that she had a firm grasp of the obvious.
DIANE

How few of us have a firm grasp of the obvious. We spend so much time rushing from one frantic moment to another that we buzz right past the obvious in our search for the exotic.

When we have a firm grasp of the obvious in our lives, we realize that it is often just that—the obvious—that gives us a feeling of serenity and calm. In fact, it is often a loss of connection with the obvious that results in our feeling off balance and not quite "with it."

What are some of the obvious things in our lives? Perhaps one of the most ignored is that our bodies are functioning. They may not be functioning perfectly and if they were not functioning at all, we would not be here. Equally obvious, we have air to breathe. The quality may be questionable, but when our lungs are needing to suck something into them, the air is waiting there, obvious, ready to come into our lungs and start the process our bodies need. There is also, obviously, water in our lives—to drink, to bathe in, to listen to, to feel, and to hold other things we like in our life, like fish and minerals. Need I go on?

We depend on many things in our life that are obvious, and yet we may not have a firm grasp of the obvious.

What are the obvious things you need to become aware of?
Let yourself notice them.

DEFINITIONS AND PRACTICAL

I need words of wisdom that are practical and everyday.

JIM

Sometimes it's necessary to revise our definition of something that we have long since believed we held firmly in place and understood. This willingness to look at and ability to change our dearly held definitions is one of the skills that we need for the continuing process of bringing our lives back into balance. Our lives are an ever-changing process and the events that impinge upon us are ever changing. This constant changing is one of the abiding realities of life. Our lives do not become balanced and stay that way. We achieve balance, growth moves to imbalance, and we return to a new balance. And so it goes with the definitions of our lives. We understand a concept one way and the changes within us and external to us often require changing definitions.

Take practicality, for example. At one stage, "practical" may mean just what we perceive to be the nuts and bolts of living, the basics, like earning money, cooking, cleaning, and sleeping. As we become more affluent, "practical" may mean the "new" necessities of life—good restaurants, expensive gifts, and trophy cars and houses. Often the spiritual things are not seen as practical. Yet as we grow internally, "things" may be seen as less important while spiritual processes and relationships may be seen as the nuts and bolts of life.

Remember, the "practical" should always be in the service of the important and "practical" is in the eye of the beholder.

Take time to sit down to write out your present definition of practical and important.

LISTENING AND TALKING

If one could only teach the English how to talk, and the Irish how to listen, society here would be quite civilized.

OSCAR WILDE

I quite agree. Rarely have two more different groups been thrown together to try to cope with one another. Yet, we can delve much deeper into this quote from the brilliant Oscar Wilde. The Irish and the English, with their difficulties with one another, can teach us a great deal about ourselves.

Recently I have had the opportunity to notice how few people truly know how to listen—actively, positively *listen*. Listening is not waiting for the other person to finish so that we can say what we want to say. Listening is not preparing what we want to say while the other is speaking. Listening is taking a deep breath and clearing ourselves so that we can be receptive to hearing what the other is saying—without interrupting. Listening is letting the words, feelings, and intuitions of the other enter into our inner space so that we have the possibility of knowing without words.

Then there is talking. When we talk, we have a sacred responsibility for everything that comes out of our mouth. We have an obligation to speak clearly, truthfully, and succinctly so that what we convey has the best possible chance to be understood. We can be somber, funny, entertaining, or serious and we are responsible for our words if we want others to listen to us.

Check out your listening and talking skills. Do you need to work on either or both? Then get at it.

FEELING OUT OF PLACE

So I didn't feel out of place because of my gender and race. I felt out of place because there were things I didn't know. It was up to me to become a sponge and learn how to take in all the information and understand it, research it, and really prepare myself for the next meeting.

CYNTHIA "COOP" COOPER

Why waste time on what others might be thinking, feeling, or projecting on us? Don't we have enough to do to keep our own side of the street clean? When we find ourselves feeling out of place, we will never feel better if we make others responsible for our feeling that way.

We feel so much better when we see what we can do to be better informed and prepared. There is always more that we can learn, more ways we can become informed, and better ways we can come to understand what is needed. If we focus on making ourselves as informed and prepared as we need to be, we won't have time to focus on others.

When all is said and done, the only person we can change is ourselves and that is enough to ask of anyone. If you continue to feel out of place, maybe you are. Accept it and move on.

When you feel out of place in a situation, immediately see what you can do to change it. What you do with yourself is key here.

HOPE

Hope sees the invisible, feels the intangible, and achieves the impossible.

ANONYMOUS

When we feel off-balance, how much we need the invisible, intangible, and impossible! In our typically human way, we respond to stress by becoming more rigid and controlling. We hold our breath and believe that if we can just grit our teeth and get through whatever it is, we can relax and get back to "normal." We focus on the visible, the tangible, and the possible, hoping to reduce our world to something manageable.

Ironically, times of stress are just when we need these nonconcretes more than ever. Just when we need hope the most, we tend to move in the opposite direction, seeing hope as a luxury we can ill afford.

At times like these, we need to stop to *remember.* If we stop for a moment, we can remember that we have been confronted with, gone through, and emerged from such situations before. Remembering can give us hope.

We need to remember that the intangible and invisible play important roles in our lives. We can count on their being there for us. We can remember that things only look impossible when we don't have all the information yet. More will come. Hope lets us know these things.

UPS AND DOWNS

The great need is for balance—when we are down, we need to get up; and when we are up, we need to remember that we have been and certainly will be again "down."

ERNEST KURTZ AND KATHERINE KETCHAM

How important memory is in our search for balance! All too often we get so enmeshed in our present state, whatever it is, that we lose all sense of perspective. We feel down and depressed, and we begin to believe that that is our only reality. We have days of joy and begin to indulge in the fantasy that life is and should be just a movement of up, up, and up, and we feel angry with and cheated by life when we slide down again. Somehow, the regular changes of life become personal attacks.

Don't despair. Life isn't attacking us. We are attacking us with our loss of memory. Our memory helps us to know at a feeling level that things will change, and that change is the truth of life. When we are down, we can remember past "downs," realize that we survived them, and look at what got us out of them. When we are "up," we can appreciate and enjoy that state and still keep our perspective.

Nurture your perspective and memory. You may even want to take some notes when you are up or down for perspective training.

PREJUDICES

Everyone is a prisoner of his own experiences. No one can eliminate prejudices—just recognize them.

EDWARD R. MURROW

Prejudice is learned. Yet it may seem so basic to our beings that we have difficulty separating it from who we are. Prejudice is also taught to us. We learn it in our homes, our schools, our churches, and our societies. It seeps into our unconscious and steals into our illusions of who we are and who others are. Prejudice removes us from our feelings of oneness with all creation, and alienating us from ourselves as well as others. Although prejudice is commonplace, it is not natural. It prevents us from moving naturally through our walk of life.

We may have racial prejudices; prejudices against women, against men, against certain nationalities, religions, social workers, tall people, fat people, young people, old people, people with money, people without money—the list goes on and on. Of course our prejudices are destructive to others and most of us fail to realize how they distort us. Prejudices distort our perceptions, our reality, and our visions. They eliminate possible friendships, learnings, and growth. They ask too much and give too little. They are a poor investment in ourselves.

As we grow, we find that we can no longer afford to keep our prejudices.

Sit down with a group of people you trust and explore prejudices—honestly. They won't vanish overnight and naming them is the first step.

SMALL ACTS WITH GREAT LOVE

We cannot do great things on this earth. We can only do small things with great love.

MOTHER TERESA

While we are waiting for great things, we may miss the opportunity for little things.

I have a neighbor who has the most wonderful grapefruit tree in the world. This tree has the juicest, sweetest grapefruit I have ever tasted. People are always wanting grafts from this tree. The morning after I have returned from a long trip, there is usually a bag or two of grapefruit on my doorstep. I not only feel loved by the gift, I feel *known*, because my neighbor knows how much I love that grapefruit. A simple act done with great love.

Often when I am baking a special dish, I make two and take one next door. Or when I receive a special treat like Christmas pears, I share them. A simple act done with great love.

The funny thing about doing small acts with great love is that we find deep in ourselves a lovingness of ourselves when we behave this way.

Most of the important acts in life are very simple.

Each day, look for the opportunity to do small things with great love. You'll be surprised at how good you feel and at how these acts spread.

ORDINARINESS

Ordinary folk, like you and me, must be greatly loved by God since there are so many of us, always have been, most likely always will be.

Sister Thérèse of Lisieux

What a funny lot we are! We expend huge globs of energy wanting to *be* somebody when we already *are* somebody. We are unique. There is no one like us, never has been, never will be. And, that's not enough for many of us. We are so fearful of being ordinary that we push ourselves, sometimes ruthlessly, sometimes absurdly, to be different. We want to stand out from the crowd. We want to be the head that sticks out above the rest (which of course means that it has the greatest possibility of being lopped off!). And yet we all have the opportunity to celebrate the unique ordinariness that is ours.

Ordinary people have such tremendous opportunities. We are greatly loved by God. That gives us something to ease into. We have the wonderful opportunity of privacy. We are not hounded by the press and the media. We can quietly drive home after our ordinary day's work, get out of our ordinary car with quiet ease, and share the evening with those we love in an activity of our choice.

Ordinariness has its advantages.

Today, let yourself bask in the glory of being ordinary. Be aware of the gifts this ordinariness offers you.

LISTENING

Someone to tell it to is one of the fundamental needs of human beings.

MILES FRANKLIN

We need someone to listen to us. Being listened to isn't just a desire; it is a basic human need. There are many people in our lives who are willing to talk to us, and even a few who are sure that they know what we need to do, yet how rare is the person who genuinely *listens*.

Often, the only people who listen to us are spouses, boyfriends/girlfriends, or partners. Talking and listening are certainly among the most important ways we approach intimacy. Yet, having only one listener in our lives can put a great burden on that relationship.

We need to round up family, friends, and partners who can listen to us. It is generally agreed that women tend to be better listeners than men. And yet men can learn when the motivation is there. (They're not dumb, you know.) It is really good if we have *both* men and women in our lives who can hear us.

Of course, listening is best done when it goes both directions.

Do a listener inventory of your family, friends, and partner. Do you have people you can talk honestly with? What (if anything) do you need to do about this?

DIARIES

That all my dreams might not prove empty, I have been writing this useless account—though I doubt it will long survive me. [Written in 1306.]

LADY NIJO

Often people find that writing in a diary adds balance to their lives.

There are as many concepts of diaries as there are blades of grass. Unfortunately, many of us give up before we begin because the task (and we too often view it as a task) seems too daunting; we worry that we don't know the *proper* way to do it.

There *is* no one, right way to keep a diary. I have a folding notepad with a built-in light and an attached pen that writes under any conditions. It's great for what I need. Some people offer pointers and they are just that—pointers. First of all, remember that if you want to embark on a diary, it is for you. It is yours. It is *only* for you. Having this one thing just for ourselves is a special experience in and of itself. Our diary can consist of our list of things to do. It can be a place for completely random thoughts and ideas that we like. It can be our secret, hidden poet coming out. It can be our hopes and dreams.

Most importantly, we need to remember that we are not a slave to our diary. We keep it because we *want* to.

During times of stress, we may want to talk through issues with ourselves in our diary. We may want a "gratitude" diary, where we jot down good events so we can savor them again and again. The possibilities are limitless.

Check out to see if you would like to experiment with a diary.

SEEING GOD—PRAYER

If you begin to live life looking for the God that is all around you, every moment becomes a prayer.

FRANK BIANCO

As I have explored my Native American ancestry, I have been amazed with the humility and serenity that I find in the "old ones." In spite of what has happened to them and to their people, I always experience a peacefulness and balance I rarely see anywhere else in "common" people (in other words, excluding the Dalai Lama and others like him). What I have come to know over the years and have begun to experience is that serenity and balance come from the very basic act of seeing God all around us.

It's really quite simple. When we look at a tree, God is there. When we look at a flower, God is there. When we look at the sky, God is there. When we look at the earth, God is there.

We can see God in the faces of people on the street, in the faces of our children, our friends, our partners, our colleagues, and our bosses. When we see God shining through the faces of all those around us—those like us and those unlike us—every moment becomes a prayer and the world becomes a different place to live in.

Practice seeing God wherever you look. See what happens within you as a result.

CURIOSITY—BOREDOM

Bored people, unless they sleep a lot, are cruel.

RENATA ADLER

Being bored is not sophisticated; it's boring.

When do we get bored? We get bored when we are not present to our lives and the world around us. Boredom signals the loss of curiosity and exploration, a loss that must be the actual process of edging toward death.

Curiosity is not just for children! Curiosity is that movement inside us that is stirred by wonder and awe and fanned by the deep knowledge that no matter how much we know, there are always new worlds to explore.

Some years ago, I went into a frame shop to have a simple print framed. I emerged two hours later having explored what seemed like a million types of glass, frames, and borders. I never knew there was so much to framing a small print! I was fascinated by the choices and felt that a whole new world had presented itself for my exploration. I painted LEARNING on the experience, not BOREDOM.

Pick out something you have been curious about this week and explore it. Curiosity is far better than cruelty.

DECISIONS

Decision is a risk rooted in the courage of being free.
PAUL TILLICH

We are very tricky in our decision-making . . . and talented and creative. When we have decisions to make, some of us will go to extreme measures to avoid making them.

Faced with a decision, we will gather data repeatedly, wanting everything to be perfectly clear. We believe that given enough information, we can be certain of our decision. We want to be *right;* we want to believe that in every situation there must be a *right* decision.

After we have gathered tons of information, we think. We think, and think, and think. We obsess; we figure different angles; we push ourselves to delineate *all* the possible consequences and outcomes. We want to be safe.

Then, if all else fails, we try to get someone else to make the decision for us. Unfortunately, there are plenty of people eager to advise us, even though most of them are quite unwilling to make their *own* decisions.

Silently and subtly we hand our power over to those who are willing to make our decisions, and we relax. However, having lost our personal power and our courage, we end up feeling uneasy with ourselves and others.

We don't have to approach decisions this way. There are other options.

Practice not giving power away on small decisions, and the big ones will fall into place. Start with something as simple as choosing foods you really like to eat or clothes you really like to wear.

FLATTERY

I hate careless flattery, the kind that exhausts you in your effort to believe it.

WILSON MIZENER

How cunning is flattery. It is like alcohol or drugs. We are born not knowing or believing that we need it and, with even a little taste of it, we easily come to the conclusion that it is one of life's little necessities. With only a slight exposure to flattery, we can turn it into a frantically sought after drug. Unfortunately, as with all obsessions, it may not be all that it seems.

What is astonishing about most good flattery (the kind we usually call compliments) is that if it is indeed "careful" flattery, we already knew it anyway. Therefore, flattery is not a surprise; it is a validation from others of something we already knew or suspected. The dependency part is when we come to believe that others have the power to validate us. *No one* has that power. Only *we* can validate ourselves.

The problem with "care*less*" flattery is that even if we know it is a con, we may slip into an attempt to delude ourselves into believing it. There's little worse and more unsettling than a double con—one in which our participation is required.

When we accept the truth about ourselves, true flattery is hearing this truth and opening ourselves to the possibility to accept it.

Check out your ability to accept compliments. Do you need some work in this area?

CHEERFULNESS

The most manifest sign of wisdom is continued cheerfulness.
MONTAIGNE

It's true, you know. The wisest people I know are almost always cheerful. This does not mean that their lives are perfect or that everything is served up to them on a silver platter. In fact, it is often quite the contrary. It is how they approach what is served up to them that makes their life cheerful, not what is served.

For example, one of my neighbors—a woman in her eighties whom I love very much—was recently hospitalized because she was getting a bit confused and forgetful. She is one of my best sources of wisdom; I learn a lot from her. When I went to visit her, she conspiratorially whispered to me, "You know, sometimes I get confused. I don't know what hospital I'm in."

I told her that I'd noticed her occasional confusion and assured her that I didn't suppose it really mattered as long as she was comfortable and content. Besides, I liked that this hospital was closer to my house. She quickly agreed and then said, "Well, you die if you worry and you die if you don't—so why worry?"

She's had a good life—not an easy one and a good one. Cheerfulness has helped a lot.

When you have an opportunity to be gloomy, switch to cheerfulness and see what happens. You may be surprised. (Phony cheerfulness won't work though. It may take a while to get to genuine cheerfulness, and keep at it until you do.)

RAISING CHILDREN

Two parents can't raise a child any more than one. You need a whole community—everybody—to raise a child.

TONI MORRISON

How difficult it is to find balance in our lives when we have small children to raise! Raising children is not just about being custodial and seeing to their health and well-being. Raising children means teaching, loving, conveying respect, opening doors of exploration, standing back and waiting, supporting only as long as necessary until they can take over, teaching the process of loving and relating, and opening the opportunity for intimacy with a range of people from many walks of life.

To believe that one or two parents can provide all this is limited and pure insanity. No wonder so many young parents feel so frantic and overextended. They are.

Children are an asset to the whole community and to the whole world. They are not just "ours" or our family's. They belong to the future, and we have the sacred opportunity to care for them and guide them for a while.

Stop and look at your children as a "sacred opportunity."
See what possibilities exist beyond the one or two parents for
helping to raise them. Children need the richness of diversity.

PEACEFUL SLEEP

Fathers, our hearts are good . . .
when we are at peace . . . we sleep easy . . .

SPOTTED TAIL

Sleep is one of the most precious gifts. A peaceful rest is often taken for granted, yet sleep is as important as food, air, and water. Without it, our bodies refuse to work properly, and a functional balance is impossible.

Sleep restores the body. Scientists tell us this, and more importantly, we know this from our experience. And that is not all sleep does.

Sleep is also a mental and a spiritual refresher. We "go to school" when we sleep. During sleep, our mind and being move to realms beyond our conscious knowing—realms where we can learn what we need to know at different levels of reality. This knowledge can help us in all areas of our lives and is especially helpful in decisions determining our next steps in living.

Sleep is also a spiritual refresher. During deep sleep we move beyond concerns of everyday life and unite with the core of our being. This uniting refreshes and restores our being and supports our spiritual path.

Sleep is magical and practical at the same time, something to be taken seriously and treated with the highest regard. Sleep is one of life's great balancers. We need to do what we can to move into it fully.

Make it a habit to do what you can to clear up your part of unresolved issues before you go to bed every night so that peaceful sleep comes. This may mean simply letting go of what you cannot change.

LEARNING FROM ADVERSITY

Barn's burnt down—now I can see the moon

MASAHIDE

Nothing is ever all bad. No matter how bad it is, there is always the possibility of good coming out of it. In the last analysis, it is what we do with a situation that defines the situation. We read about a wife and mother whose husband and children are killed in an accident. She, of course, is devastated, and yet she goes on to become an astute and successful businesswoman as she takes over the family business, using her grief to heal herself and the business at the same time.

Or we hear about a friend who was passed over for a promotion and was sure his life was ended. Yet, this experience pushed him out of a company where he felt uneasy and forced him to start up a business that expressed his spirituality. And he became happily successful.

Often we hear "God does for us what we cannot do for ourselves."

Sometimes "God's nudge" is not what we would have asked for, and yet maybe it is what is needed to help us truly enjoy the moon.

Go look at the moon and see if any obstructing "barns" you have built come into your awareness.

EXERCISE

I am persuaded that the greater part of our complaints arise from want of exercise.

MARIE DE RABUTIN-CHANTAL, MARQUISE DE SÉVENGÉ

Exercise—working out—getting in shape—reducing stress—going for the burn—striving for endorphins—no pain, no gain . . .

Where did we ever get the idea that torture by others isn't okay, and self-torture is? Torture is torture.

Busy people who do too much don't have time for gradual changes. We want everything at once.

Exercise is good for us. There's no doubt about it. Exercise that is pleasurable and soothes the soul is even better for us. Our bodies don't exist in isolation. They are we and we are they. The best exercise we can do is one that relaxes and feeds all parts of our being while helping to keep our bodies healthy.

All too often, we don't exercise because we haven't taken the time to find out what really fits for us. We approach exercise like we do so many other things—as something we have to do that's good for us, something we need to finish. No wonder we avoid it when we can.

Take the time to explore exercise modalities—stretching, aerobics, walking, workouts, running. See what works for you, remembering that preferences and needs may change.

Be kind to yourself.

FEELINGS

Our feelings are our most genuine paths to knowledge.
AUDRE LORDE

Let's hear it for feelings!

Feelings are the doors through which we have to go to reach beyond ourselves. Many of us have been taught that we can't trust our feelings, and this has thrown us out of balance with ourselves and with our connection with our spirituality. We cannot reach our spirituality through our minds. The mind "thinks about" the spiritual, whereas our feelings "experience" the spiritual. Both our minds and our feelings enrich our knowledge of our spiritual selves. We *can* reach spirituality with our feelings alone. Our minds by themselves can only find abstract concepts.

If we spent as much time enriching our feelings and our awareness of relationship with them as we do enriching our minds, imagine what might happen!

Start working with your feelings. Honor them. When you feel something, notice it; assume that it is there for a very good reason and let yourself truly feel it. Start to notice those small tinges that are the precursors to full-fledged feelings.

Remember, busy people are "feeling challenged."

FEELING GOOD

I just wanta feel good.

ANONYMOUS

There's nothing wrong with feeling good. In fact, feeling good is a gift of being human. It's the paths we choose to feeling good that sometimes get us into trouble.

We will never feel good if we try to do it at someone else's expense. As Dr. Seuss's *Yertle the Turtle* illustrates, we will never feel good about getting to the top if we have to crush and destroy others to get there. Also, we don't really like ourselves when we try to look good by making someone else feel bad. Eventually that truth-speaker inside of us breaks through our well-constructed wall of denial and lets us know that we don't feel that good about ourselves or what we have done.

It's okay to be honest about the things in which we excel, and yet when that slips into boasting and bragging, something inside us, however subtle, sounds an alarm.

It's funny how human beings are constructed. We almost always feel best about ourselves when we are doing something for someone else, contributing to the greater good, or just being sensitive. And, if we do something *just* so we will feel good about ourselves, it rarely works. We may have to do some practice runs before we get it.

Start with simple gestures: say hello; do little things; be of service whenever you can. Feeling good is not as difficult as it may seem.

FAREWELLS

Every arrival foretells a leave-taking: every birth a death. Yet each death and departure comes to us as a surprise, a sorrow neveranticipated. Life is a long series of farewells; only the circumstances should surprise us.

JESSAMYN WEST

Perhaps one of the most important skills we can develop as a human being is learning to do graceful farewells. We have so much resistance to accepting the obvious fact that "life is a long series of farewells." We want permanence. We want stasis. We want security. And we believe, deep in our souls, that security is definitely related to and dependent upon permanence and stasis. We look to the hills and we look to the old trees to teach us about permanence and stasis, failing to see that they are slowly and imperceptibly disintegrating and changing and teaching us about farewells. We put our faith in manmade structures, hoping for proof that permanence is possible, and they let us down.

With stubborn insistence, we demand constants. With unrelenting precision, our demands are thwarted. To rile against reality is futile.

Instead, we can spend our time learning to deal gracefully with change. Change is our given. We are always saying farewell—to a favorite cup newly broken, at the end of a telephone conversation, as relationships and friendships wane, or to cars we love. We may maintain our right to be surprised by the circumstances, and we can grow into the beauty of graceful farewells.

Practice graceful farewelling.

QUICK FIXES

It was so cold I almost got married.

SHELLEY WINTERS

One of the ways we unbalance ourselves is to settle for a quick, easy fix instead of dealing with the real issues that are troubling us. When we are busy, we lunge for the quick relief (a candy bar, a drink, a marriage, a new job), when in the long run, the relief may just compound the problem. That's the problem with rushing into a solution. Real solutions usually take time to discover. Quick fixes add more problems than they solve.

Although our lives tend to be lived at a fast pace, important problems and solutions just do not bend easily to that agenda. Indeed, maybe that is the importance of the big problems: perhaps they are in our lives to teach us the process of waiting for the clarity of a "right" solution.

If something is important, that issue is worth taking the time to sit with, to pray about, to talk over with people we trust, and to act on in a way that is sane for us.

We are always worth the time it takes to come to a solution to the real problem.

Whenever you want to jump to the quick fix, see the urge as a signal that there may be something important underneath and give yourself the willingness to see it.

GOD

Those who've never rebelled against God or at some point in their lives shaken their fists in the face of heaven, have never encountered God at all.

CATHERINE MARSHALL

God is much too complex not to struggle with. Part of our humanness lies in wanting to reduce God down to concepts, ideas, and experiences that we can handle. That's somewhat like trying to squeeze a champion sumo wrestler into a pair of size-small, control-top pantyhose. Good luck.

Our minds just don't handle God very well.

God seems much easier with our beings, our hopes, our dreams, our wonder, and our participation. Most of all, I believe God loves our participation.

This means that struggling often wins out over holiness, and mistakes over correctness. Sometimes, I have come to believe, that God just wants a good laugh, and there is nothing like a bunch of humans to provide it.

Think of God roaring with laughter as you try to control your little universe, and you'll have more fun.

USEFUL LIVING

I believe that any man's life will be filled with constant, unexpected encouragements . . . if he makes up his mind to do his level best each day of his life—that is, tries to make each day reach as nearly as possible the high water mark of pure, unselfish, useful living.

BOOKER T. WASHINGTON

When we get too busy for useful living, we are in trouble. We may be rushing around looking very busy. We may be over-burdened, overworked, and overextended, and, are we useful? Is what we are doing useful? Is it useful to us? Is it useful to someone else? The lowest-paid, lowest-prestige job can be very useful, while the top-executive position can be set up in such a way as to be utterly useless. When our experience of our work is that it contributes to useful living, no matter what it is we feel good about ourselves.

When we get frantic and do too much, we lose sight of meaning. Under these circumstances, the doing replaces the meaning. The job suffers, and we suffer. We get caught up in a cycle of doing for doing's sake, and the importance of making a contribution gets lost.

At times like these, we need to stop, take stock, and reexamine what we are doing. Try to remember why we started this work in the first place; think back on times when we believed in what we were doing. Meaning and useful living are essential elements of our path to balance.

FRANTIC—CHOICES—
OVERREACTING

Rushing, frantic, panic—it took me a long time to realize that these are not necessarily the way life is.

ANONYMOUS

Where did we get the idea that we have to live life as an emergency? We have developed the idea that to be alive, we have to face one drama after another. We overreact, blow things completely out of proportion and get irritated, confused, annoyed, and negative. We let little, teeny things bother us, blowing them completely out of proportion.

Whoa, stop; wait a minute! Whew—take a breath. We're not in an adrenaline-ridden movie!

I recently saw a movie in which the lead rarely, unless drunk, spoke below a scream. The background music was relentless heavy rock, and the scenes were filled with sounds of bodies crushing against one another on the gridiron. At the end we just sat there, silent, completely exhausted and drained, almost unable to get up after having paid a tidy sum for this experience. Does art (and I use the term loosely!) imitate life, does life imitate life, or is there no relationship?

Ultimately, it all boils down to choices. When we see that we are not at the mercy of frantic and panic, that how we relate to our lives greatly influences what our lives are and become, and that overreaction results in frustration, we have a chance for something else.

Look at the way you approach your problems. Do you over react? Try stepping back, taking a few deep breaths, and giving yourself some time. Remember—when in doubt, don't.

HUMOR AS A BALANCER

Humor is reason gone mad.

GROUCHO MARX

That's right! How well put. And there are times when it is *necessary* for reason to go mad. A little reasonableness, like many things, is very good. Too much reasonableness can become stagnating and stifling.

Let's not knock reasonableness. It's great when performing surgery, figuring income tax, and teaching quantum physics (and there must be other good examples of where reasonableness is most appropriate). Unfortunately, whenever I think of one, a humorous idea creeps in, asking this one to be eliminated. Take funerals, for example. Surely we need to be reasonable at funerals. Then I remember my father's, where the memorial service started out on a very somber tone. Then we started telling "Daddy stories" that set us to laughing and crying together. I think my father would have enjoyed it (and probably did). We certainly did.

Humor is not irreverence. It is the balancing component with reason that makes the complexities of life seem ultimately sensible.

What is your humor quotient? Have you become overly serious? Try laughing at yourself and your most serious moods and see what happens.

WHAT IS REAL

And they believe that what they are doing is real.

PETE

The above phrase was uttered by a friend of mine as we drove down a street in Sydney, Australia. We were right in the middle of a downtown area, surrounded by high-rise office buildings. We had just come down from the Blue Mountains and were feeling a bit overwhelmed by the city. I had just said that I didn't think I could stand working in one of those buildings, when people began to pour out by the hundreds for their lunch break. That's when Pete said, "And they believe that what they are doing is real."

This phrase stuck with me, and I have pondered it often. I have long since come to the awareness that one of the areas on which we tend to put our main focus—money—is not real. Money is something conceived of and made up by human beings. It is legal tender. It is not real. Native people have asked, "Can you eat it? Can you build with it? Can it keep you warm?" It's not real. Yet, much of our time is spent dealing with it.

Then I began to look at other issues from the same perspective. When I get very upset with someone about what seems like a life-and-death issue, when I stop and back off, I can then ask myself the question, "Is it real?" Often the answer is "no."

When we stop to ask ourselves whether getting just the right lamp to fit with our decor or winning the debate on a major corporate decision is real, scarily the answer may be no.

The next time you get worked up about something, stop to ask whether the issue is real or not.

ATTITUDES

No life is so hard that you can't make it easier by the way you take it.

ELLEN GLASGOW

Sometimes we get almost dizzy with the power we have! We have the power to make our life easier just by how we approach it. What a revolutionary thought!

Life is a process in which we can participate, stand back and bemoan our fate, or we can try to ignore it and get through it as best we can. The decision is ours. We can make life much more difficult with the decisions we make, or we can make it easier.

One of the ways we make our life hard is by convincing ourselves that we are a victim. Victims don't have much fun. We may have been victimized in many different ways and it is up to us whether we become a victim or not. I may not like what others do to me. I may not like my station in life. I may not like what life has dealt me. Yet, no one but I myself can take the next step and make me a victim. Victims are unhappy and resentful, miserable and isolated. Isn't it great to know that we have a choice?

Check out situations where you feel like a victim and see if you can change your attitude about each of them.

POSITIVES

I try to turn everything into a positive.
CYNTHIA "COOP" COOPER

Whatever happens to us, for us, or against us, in the end it is what we do with the experience that makes it what it is.

Several years ago I was threatened with what to me was a horrible lawsuit (having had no experience with that kind of legal thing before). It was so off the wall and seemed so unfair to me that I was instantly furious. My first thought was, "I don't believe it. I'll get that so-and-so." As quickly as that thought had come, another more important one followed on its heels and sent me reeling. I instantly knew what my task was in this process. It came to me as clear as a bell that my learning in this process was to stay away from the victim-perpetrator dualism. Since I believe that those who see themselves as victims become perpetrators and that all perpetrators have seen themselves as victims, this was very important.

For example, I had immediately felt like an innocent victim and so had instantly become a perpetrator. I wanted to "get" that person. My spiritual self quickly intervened, showing me that regardless of the outcome, my role was not to become a victim *or* a perpetrator. When I saw what my task was to be, the rest fell into place.

Never have I been so tested not to let myself become victim or a perpetrator. It was a good learning.

We've heard a lot about turning lemons into lemonade. How about turning everything into a positive today and seeing what the learning is for you?

THE EARTH

It is a wholesome and necessary thing for us to turn again to the earth and in the contemplation of her beauties to know the sense of wonder and humility.

RACHEL CARSON

Both wonder and humility take time. And, our wonder and humility toward the earth may take some time and focus, indeed.

We have taken the earth for granted for a long time. As a result, getting back to a consciousness in our relationship with the earth is not always easy. The problems of pollution, toxic waste, and unsafe and destroyed land seem so overwhelming that we just don't know where to begin.

How about starting with ourselves?

What happens to a seed when it is put into the ground? It sprouts and grows. Can we *hold* a seed and make it grow? I think not. We can look at every weed and flower and see a miracle in progress. We *can* return to wonder. The earth holds so many wonders that even when we have some understanding of the processes (like how oil or diamonds are made) we can experience great wonder if we only let ourselves feel it.

With wonder comes humility. Ultimately the earth puts us in our place. The earth feeds, clothes, houses, and sustains us. That's just a fact. We feel wonder and humility when we recognize and acknowledge this fact.

Where are your wonder and humility toward the earth? Start where you are and see what these two traits contribute toward environmentalism in you.

TALKING

Most of my Indian friends were of the opinion that talking, unless wisely and frugally done, causes one's power to leak away, reducing him to being just another unnecessary noise.

J. ALLEN BOONE

It's really hard to get it right. We're told we have to be assertive and put ourselves out there to get anywhere in this world, and then J. Allen Boone tells us that talking unwisely and unfrugally can drain our power away. What's a person to do?

Learning the power of active silence is an art well worth the time it takes to learn it. Have you ever been in a group of people where everyone was just chattering away, trying to be seen and get their point across when the words of one previously silent person left the others speechless?

Perhaps our power does leak out when our focus is not where it should be. When we talk wisely and frugally, we don't have much to say, *so* every word counts. When our silence is confused, self-centered, or controlling, we have little to add. When we give our power away by focusing on others, we leak power.

We can learn ways of participating in silence and ways of being meaningful when we speak. None of us wants to be an "unnecessary noise," and each of us has that potential.

See what you have to learn about talking wisely and frugally. Are there ways you leak your power through talking?

FREEDOM—RESPONSIBILITY

Man is condemned to be free; because once thrown into the world, he is responsible for everything he does.

JEAN PAUL SARTRE

Freedom and responsibility—the words seem to go together. We cannot have freedom unless we are willing to take responsibility for our lives, and it is through the act of taking responsibility that we begin to feel a sense of power and freedom.

It almost seems that modern psychology has so convinced us that we are victims that we are willing to throw out the baby with the bathwater, giving up the potential of freedom in order not to have to take responsibility. What a loss!

Responsibility is not about accountability or blame. Accountability and blame are much too small to encompass responsibility. Accountability and blame have distorted our concept of responsibility.

We are not responsible for events we did not cause and cannot control. We *are* responsible for what we say and do and how we react to happenings that are out of our control. That's plenty; that's enough.

Try freedom. Try responsibility. You might like them.

Spend one day being utterly responsible for everything you do. Feel the return of your personal power and freedom.

SINGING YOUR SONG

And those who want to sing will find a song.

ANONYMOUS

Our songs can be almost anything we want them to be.

Knowing that we really want to sing is the first step. Throughout history, sages have told us how powerful a force intention is. Novels, movies, and great stories often revolve around some person who knew that they really wanted something enough to go after it.

The song we choose and the finding of it are very important. And the journey along the way can make the song so much sweeter when it is finally sung.

We need to remember that every step of our journey is incorporated into the final song. If we step on others to get our song, we will have sour notes. If we disregard ourselves and our needs in the process of composing our song, we will have discordant tones. If we do not take notice of the alternative paths along our way, we will not gather the right harmonies for the full song.

If our movement toward the song is filled with sharing love with those we meet, seeing ourselves participating in a process and nurturing that process, and being open to codas and new directions, our song will be filled with richness, harmony, and joy.

Trust that you have a song to sing and that you will find it.

LEARNING AND TEACHERS

How we learn is what we learn.

BONNIE FRIEDMAN

Today may be one of those days when our world begins to shift toward a new kind of balance.

We all have teachers in our lives, and we all *need* teachers in our lives. The teachers are always there. What we learn from them is up to us. Our ability to identify the teacher and to learn is directly related to how open-minded we are and the attitude with which we approach everyone and everything that comes into our sphere. When we see all people and things as potential teachers, we have taken a great leap toward balance. This attitude requires, of course, that we be able to see that everyone and everything has some knowledge that we don't have.

I met a tree recently who started out as a rather sickly houseplant. Some unknowing person had planted it in a very unlikely place, considering the kind of plant it is. In spite of all the disadvantages put in its way, however, that tree has focused its attention on growing. It has grown and grown, becoming a majestic, heavy-rooted banyan tree. Every time I look at that tree, I see how I let obstacles get in my way. That tree knows more than I do about growing.

Today, start developing an attitude that everyone and everything you meet has something to teach you that you don't know. Approach the world as filled with teachers—some of whom you may not like or want to emulate.

WRITING

For me, writing something down was the only road out.
ANNE TYLER

All of us are writers.

We may not become *famous* writers and we are still writers.

Few things are as soothing as putting pen to paper (or fingers to keyboard, for some). Simply writing something down gives it new meaning, and yet writing is much more than that. The very act of writing releases unbalanced energies and lets them flow out of our bodies, where they blossom into fireflies as they hit the atmosphere.

We stop ourselves from writing with all kinds of self-imposed gimmicks and untruths. "I'm not a *good* writer." (Who cares and who said we had to be good writers and who defines good writers anyway?) "I need to have a purpose for writing; I need to know how it is going to be used." (Bull. Writing has its own intrinsic value as a process in which we engage and become engaged; it doesn't have to go anywhere!) "I don't know *how* to write." (Many famous writers invented a style that then became *the* way to do it.)

So why stop ourselves? It's the process of writing that's important.

Pick out a good pen (I love space pens myself—they write under any conditions), get a pad or a notebook ready or engage that laptop. It's time to get started! Even lists can soothe.

PATTERNS OF LIFE

All is pattern, all life, but we can't always see the pattern when we're part of it.

BELVA PLAIN

Often, we are so busy participating in life that we never step back to look at the larger picture. Even more often, we have set up our lives at such a hectic pace and are so overextended that we are not actually participating in life. We are being *driven* by a life that we have constructed in such a way as to be sure to miss out on what life is *really* about.

No matter who we are or how we live our lives, all of us can benefit from taking some time to stop, back off from busyness, and perceive our lives from a larger perspective.

We don't have time, you say? Nonsense! We can *take* the time. That choice is always ours. We need times when we can disengage for a day, a week, or a month to get an eagle-eye view of what we are doing and what we are all about. Living consciously is one of the greatest gifts we can give ourselves.

Periodically, set aside some time for yourself and tell your inner being that you are ready to see the patterns you are living and not living. The information, which may come in thoughts, dreams, intuitions, or noticings, is a great balancer.

WOUNDS—COURAGE

Do you suppose if a wound goes real deep, the healing of it can hurt almost as bad as what caused it?

LEE DAVID ZLOTOFF IN *THE SPITFIRE GRILL*

Very few, if any, of us do not carry around old wounds from our childhood and our more recent past. These wounds and experiences are the learning opportunities of our lives.

Frequently, we want to romanticize wounds, indulging in the belief that some wounds cannot be healed. This is just not true. All wounds, no matter how painful, can be healed. We have only to be willing to go through the deep process of healing, no matter what is required.

The lovely thing about our inner being is that we have to reach a certain level of maturity, strength, and awareness before it will bring up these old wounds and memories. The very fact that they are coming up is an indicator of how far we have come.

When we stand back and look at this issue of old wounds, it is like looking at the difference between chronic pain and the pain of childbirth. Chronic pain hurts and hurts and goes on and on. Childbirth *really* hurts, *and* yet there is something to show for it when it's over.

Only one caution—never, never try to force (or let someone, else force) your old pain to come up. Deal with it as it comes up in the process of life, and make sure you have a safe, supportive, noninterfering environment in which to go through it.

Develop an attitude that old wounds can be healed, and see what happens.

TOURISTS

Prayer for many is like a foreign land. When we go there, we go as tourists. Like most tourists, we feel uncomfortable and out of place. Like most tourists, we therefore move on before too long and go somewhere else.

ROBERT MCAFEE BROWN

We visit so many of the important aspects of life as tourists! We go from one relationship to another as if trying to find the perfect hotel. We find that we can recommend some aspects of many hotels, and yet none is quite perfect.

We visit various landscapes and see the beauty and majesty of each wonderful place. Yet, we don't have to take the time to learn to live with it. We are like the tourists who visit Hawaii, exhilarated by the glorious lushness and greenery and yet upset if it rains during "their week" there.

We know how to be tourists. Do we know how to be residents in our lives?

What would a commitment to your form of prayer look like? Try it.

RESPONSIBILITY FOR OUR MOUTHS

I don't let my mouth say nothin' my head can't stand.
LOUIS ARMSTRONG

It's important that our mouths be connected to our brains!

Part of learning to live in balance is learning that we are responsible for what comes out of our mouths. Some of us have learned that we are responsible for what goes *into* our mouths. (Well, maybe we have not *quite* learned that we are responsible for what goes into our mouths and how we are affected by what we ingest. And, we may have begun to *toy* with the concept.)

Many of us are even slower to get the idea that we are responsible for what comes *out* of our mouth. We pride ourselves on "saying what we think," even if our thoughts are not clear. All too often we experience that our mouths open and words just come tumbling out. Sometimes we have an audience, get on a roll, and are willing to push the limits just to get a laugh, even if it is at someone else's expense. Or we may find ourselves talking like an expert about something about which we have very little knowledge, and we do not know how to gracefully extricate ourselves. Then we have the experience of wanting to reach out into the air in front of us to push words that are hanging there in space back into our mouths.

Relax. It takes a while to learn that we are responsible for what comes out of our mouths and even longer to assume responsibility. However, the learning is worth it.

Are there words you have put out there that you need to do something about? Go do whatever you need to do to return to balance.

DIFFERENCES AND SAMENESS

Everything the same; everything distinct.

ZEN PROVERB

Did you ever consider that one of our major tasks in life is to realize our sameness *and* our distinctness?

All too often, we set up our sameness and our distinctness as a dualism. We trick ourselves into believing that if we are similar to others, sharing values and visions, that all distinctness will disappear. Or we focus on our singularity and slowly slide into the abyss of "terminal uniqueness." Terminal sameness and terminal uniqueness are equally deadly, especially when we flop back and forth between the two of them.

There are other options!

When we, in the depth of our being, know and experience the beautiful oneness of all creation, we feel the peace and security of an interconnectedness that goes completely beyond our understanding. There is a belongingness that informs all our being and doing and brings balance to our lives.

Yet, within this oneness, this connectedness, is a distinctness, a uniqueness that gives us our definition. And, with this definition, we know that we must make our contribution to the world; no one else can make it for us. We have a unique responsibility to the universe.

Knowing the truths of sameness and distinctness gives us balance for living.

Today, look around you and see the sameness between you and others, even the others you don't like or with whom you feel uncomfortable.

DOING RIGHT

Always do right! This will gratify some people and astonish the rest.

MARK TWAIN

What a concept: to gratify and astonish by doing right! We have been led to believe that we can gratify by breaking our backs to take care of people and that we can astonish by being outlandish, neither of which adds greatly to our feelings of internal balance and serenity.

Doing what is right for us seems so much more of a challenge. First we must determine what for us is "right action" (to borrow from the Zen concept of "right living"—a concept I love). Right action is not an abstract concept. It is a practical act of living that involves acting and doing. When we know what is right action for us, we have to be willing to exert the courage necessary to carry it out, especially if it may damage our "nice person" image. Then, we have to be willing to deal with the not always positive and often astonished responses. Quite an order—*and* it can be fun! In fact, doing right can be more fun than anything in the world, and it gives us a sense of integrity and freedom in the process.

Think of instances when you have done the right thing. How did you feel? You might want to try doing it again!

GUILT

Many people feel "guilty" about things they shouldn't feel guilty about, in order to shut out feelings of guilt about things they should feel guilty about.

SYDNEY J. HARRIS

Guilt has been getting a bad rap in modern circles. There's nothing wrong with guilt. In fact, guilt can be a very appropriate response to having done something we know is wrong. It's what we *do* with guilt that makes it a problem, not guilt itself.

When we do something that we know (or come to know) does not fit into our belief system or something that we know is harmful to ourselves or others, or we know we should not have done, guilt is an appropriate response from our inner beings. It is *appropriate* that we feel bad about what we have done. These feelings of guilt can serve the very good purpose of being an activator to owning our behavior, making our amends, and moving on with our lives, all the wiser for our learnings.

Indulging in guilt, on the other hand, can throw us and our lives out of balance. Indulging in guilt can be a massive, never-ending, self-centered process that serves no one. Guilt indulgence can only dig us in deeper. There's no learning that emerges.

Are you hiding from some guilt that you need to feel or indulging in some guilt that you deserve to feel? Clean it up.

CHILDREN AND MEMORIES

You never know when you're making a memory.
RICKIE LEE JONES

Notice that Jones did not say *"contriving* a memory." And yet that is what we often try to do. Unfortunately, we unbalance our lives when we try to plan and manipulate a "memory moment"! Yet, if each of us stopped to let ourselves bask in memories, we would probably find out very quickly that the memories we cherish were *given* to us, not *contrived* by us.

Sometimes we try so hard to be good parents for our children that we go to great lengths to provide them with a "memory moment." We get so wound up in details and deliberations, plans and priorities, and extravagances and excitements that no one is actually able to be present for the event. It's like staging a lavish party and forgetting to send the invitations to the guests.

Sit with yourself for a while and let your memory bank spew out its contents. You may find that the richest memories involve shared experiences of living. Shared living is what balances our lives with our children, with ourselves, and with each other.

Indulge in a "memory bath." It can relax, clarify, and heal.

BALANCING ACTS
AND LIVING IN BALANCE

A balancing act is different from living in balance.

ANONYMOUS

The idea of balancing our hectic lives is much different than learning to live in balance. A balancing act is much like life on a high wire, where one false step or leaning too far in one direction can lead to disaster. Some of us have designed our lives so tightly that any change or emergency can throw us into disaster mode. For example, we have set up child care so that we deliver the children every morning and then pick them up after work. We carefully plan our work to fit into these child-care routines. Then one child gets sick or we have a special project at work and lives and households careen into a shambles. Life has knocked our balancing pole out of our hands.

Yet, that's the way life is. Life is an ever-changing process. When we try to treat it like a series of events, we will always run into trouble. The secret to living in balance is internal, not external. Living in balance can never be accomplished through the manipulation of external events.

Become more aware of what contributes to an internal feeling of balance for you.

GREAT HEARTS

We're a great heart people.

PEARL BAILEY

"A great heart people"—What an enviable label. When we get too busy, one of the first things we forget is to let ourselves be led by our heart in the important aspects of our lives.

Our brains are fine. In fact, they are even great *and* they don't really function too well without the balancing of our hearts, our feelings, and our intuitions. We need our hearts to balance our heads; and neither is as powerful as it can be without our feelings and intuitions. The truly wise and happy person is one who is balanced in the use of all four (and more!) of these aspects of our beings.

Having a *great* heart is even more important. A great heart is open to all; it expects the richness of diversity to bring excitement and new learnings, and it flows with loving and caring to all who come within its sphere.

Unfortunately, because of the recent emphasis on rational, logical thinking, some of us have become convinced that leading with the heart is dangerous, even bad. *Not so!* We may even have come to believe that our hearts have shrunk, that we no longer have the capacity to have a "great heart." *Not so!*

Experiment with having an open and great heart today and see what happens.

THE EARTH—MATERIALISM

That is the way with us Indians, goods and earth are not equal. Goods are for using on the earth.

YELLOW SERPENT

When we are thinking about balance, we usually know, at some level, that we need to consider the earth and all of nature. Yet, the challenge of bringing a contaminated and depleted earth back into balance often seems so overwhelming that we helplessly throw up our hands and keep doing what we have always done.

Perhaps we can approach this issue from a perspective that makes it easier to handle. We need to separate our goods and our materialism from the earth and its well-being. We need to become more aware of the difference between what we need and what we want, asking ourselves that question each time we start to buy goods. We can still buy things we don't need that we want *and* our awareness will have changed.

We can look at the earth as separate from things and our materialistic urges. We can begin to see the earth as a living, moving process that makes the use of goods and even our *life* and the lives of those who follow us, possible. We can begin to see the earth as separate from and important to ourselves while at the same time intimately connected in oneness with us. When we are no longer willing to do harm to ourselves, we will no longer be willing to do harm to the earth.

Sit down and take a look at the hold materialism has on you. List three ways you can live more lovingly on the earth.

POLITENESS SLIPPAGE

Be polite. Perhaps your family won't mind if you practice on them.
MINNA THOMAS ANTRIM

In our attempts to be candid, honest, forthright, straightforward, assertive, and powerful, we may have, just *may* have, forgotten how important it is to be polite.

How often when we are busily working on a task or pushing to meet a deadline do we forget to be polite along the way? We ignore the fact that without a lot of other helping hands and support we would not have been able to complete the task. We bark orders instead of saying "Would you please . . . ?" or "Do you mind getting . . . ?" or "Thank you for your help."

When we have "politeness slippage," we tend to start with those nearest and dearest to us, expecting them to be the most forgiving and understanding. We fail to realize that these are the very people whose support we need the most and who will most dearly pay the price for our slippage. A simple "Thank you" or "I appreciate that" can go a long way toward oiling a mechanism that is slipping out of balance.

Check out your "politeness slippage." You might want to start your investigation at home.

DREAMS

Dreams say what they mean, but they don't say it in daytime language.

GAIL GODWIN

Dreams add balance to our lives. There are two major kinds of dreams, and both are important.

Some dreams are hopes and wishes. Many of these were formed or discovered in childhood, and they give our forward movement a structure and focus throughout life. They may have had the rough edges knocked off over the years, and if we view them tenderly, we will see that many of them have served as wise guideposts, pointing our way whether we realized it or not at the time.

Then there are the dreams that come to us in our sleep and in near-sleeping states. These dreams are messages and experiences that our rational, logical mind does not know how to handle. Our dreams are our inner being's attempt to bypass our rational mind with our deeper feelings, instincts and spirituality. We need to let the feelings and the messages of these dreams filter deep into us so that we can integrate our wholeness. Interpretation of dreams may not be useful at all. Instead we need to "feel" into the knowing.

Honor your dreams, waking and sleeping. Respect the information they have for you.

WHAT WE WANT

I've learned to focus on what I do want and not spend time on what I don't want.

SUSAN

So many of us have spent much of our lives getting clear about what we don't want. As children, perhaps we were not really given the option of determining what we wanted or didn't want. Going through our schooling and training often was not much different, so when we finally got out on our own we gave ourselves permission to attend to what we didn't want. It's important to know what we don't want and our time spent learning that is valuable. Yet, why is it that we always find it easier to determine what we don't want than what we *do* want?

That's the tough one. What *do* we want? What do we like to wear? What do we like to eat? What results in our feeling good? What kind of living space do we want? What kinds of things around us give us peace and pleasure—art, plants, fish, animals, cushy places to flop? Do we need a place that is just ours? A room of our own that is our world may be just what we need.

Develop a growing awareness of what you do want and need and see how you can make this happen.

BEING STILL

You must learn to be still in the midst of activity, and to be vibrantly alive in repose.

INDIRA GANDHI

For people who do too much and feel out of balance, learning "to be still in the midst of activity" is key. For most of us, it's not just the activity around us that is the problem; the activity inside us is equally important. In truth, once we get a handle on the activity within us, the activity on the outside takes on less significance.

What can we do to quiet ourselves in the midst of activity?

1. *We can stop to take some deep breaths. Taking the air in slowly and letting it out slowly, honoring the pause inbetween.*

2. *We can focus our attention on our breathing, letting our minds clear.*

3. *We can take our minds off the little things that don't matter. (Most things matter a lot less than we think they do.)*

4. *We can be alert to signals that stress is building and slow down.*

5. *We can focus on our sense of gratitude for those things that are going well. (There are always more than we realize when we are feeling frantic.)*

6. *We can turn it all over to God, fate, or a power greater than ourselves and then relax.*

When the world outside and inside gets to be too much, try some or all of the above suggestions.

PROBLEMS

Problems, unfortunately, can be addicting. Like it or not, we take a certain amount of pride in the very problems that distress us.

ELOISE RISTAD

We humans are strange creatures—and lovable, I might add. What kind of beings would take pride in the very things that are giving them the most trouble—problems that they probably created themselves? Humans!

What kind of beings feel so uneasy when everything is going absolutely wonderfully that they will create a crisis just so that they can relax? Humans!

What kind of beings feel much more comfortable handling a crisis than handling ordinary peacefulness? Humans!

Is it just that we need to keep ourselves busy so we won't get into even more trouble? Do we feel more secure when we are handling crises that we have created because then we can at least have the illusion of control? Self-created problems are still problems.

Do we really need that much adrenaline?

See what problems you seem to be attached to. Are you willing to back off and let them solve themselves? Allow your mind to discover the solution while you are focusing on something else.

EXPLORING OUR INNER WONDERS

The scientist was only one side of me. I had always felt deeply connected with my other grandmother as well. My mother's mother, Alexandra, did not have much education, but when I was a child she had seemed the wisest person in the world to me.

OLGA KHARITIDI

What hidden parts of us lurk in our heritage and our DNA? Balance involves all parts of ourselves, even those parts that go beyond ourselves.

So often we get a little glimpse of aspects of ourselves that aren't completely conscious. We're at the bookstore, say, and a book that we wouldn't usually have considered looking at catches our eye. We see a show on TV, and it sparks a forgotten longing. We see an announcement in the paper of a lecture, and we feel a surprising interest.

All of these may be your inner being's way of saying "Yoohoo—I'm in here, and these are parts of you too."

We are so much more than we think we are, and we can be even more than we imagine.

Learn to trust the whisperings of your inner being to explore parts of yourself heretofore unknown—and hold on to your hat!

SOLITUDE

Solitude is more expensive these days than a Rolex watch.
ANONYMOUS

Solitude seems so much fuller than alone time. It has the added elements of peace and time. Busy mothers can get alone time, and yet they would open a vein for solitude.

Solitude gives us time to let our hair down and see what we need, do what we need, and have the quiet to explore its benefits. When we have alone time, we can take a quiet bath. When we have solitude, we can use the quiet bath to explore what we need to do with our solitude.

Busy people may be able to squeeze in alone time now and again. And people who are living in balance require solitude.

Solitude is that quiet mist of peacefulness that enters our ears and makes its own music, enters our eyes and creates its own art, and enters our pores and imagines its own muse. Solitude returns us to ourselves while expanding us beyond our boundaries.

Solitude is precious and essential.

Alone time is fine, and do you also give yourself time for solitude?

PERSEVERANCE

Great works are performed, not by strength, but by perseverance.
SAMUEL JOHNSON

It's very difficult to persevere and rush at the same time. People who do too much usually prefer to rush. Of course, we can persevere in our rushing, which we may choose to do, and then, unfortunately, we usually don't get the rewards of genuine perseverance. So what's a body to do?

We need to distinguish between perseverance—hanging in there—and holding on.

So often our holding on is related to something that has already passed. It's over and done with, and yet we don't want it to be over. We exert our will to hold on, often with disastrous results.

When we hang in there, we stick with a situation or person for as long the situation or the person requires it. Our hanging-in behavior is appropriate and related to the situation; it is not just self-will or stubbornness.

Perseverance is continuing to work at something for as long as there is value in working at it. Perseverance is being appropriately related to ourselves, the situation, and others involved. It is the commitment to seeing something through to completion and the ability to recognize when that completion has been reached.

Can you distinguish among holding on, hanging in, and perseverance in the way you function? See which elements are most balancing for you.

SELFISHNESS

Selfishness is not living as one wishes to live, it is asking others to live as one wishes to live.

RUTH RENDELL

Sometimes we just don't realize what we are doing. We don't consciously set out to be selfish. We just do our own thing. If we don't take care of number one, who will? We may even see ourselves as a very considerate person and yet still be living selfishly.

For example, when we make decisions for people who are perfectly capable of making decisions for themselves, we are being selfish. When we fill the air with cigarette smoke or pollution, we are being selfish. When we do things for people that they don't particularly *want* done for them (because we feel good about ourselves when we do it), we are being selfish. When we make noise, have kids, or play rock music around those who don't want this, we are being selfish. When we impose ideas, decisions, or beliefs, we are being selfish.

Selfishness is much more subtle than we would like to believe and much more prevalent than we would hope.

Take a good, hard look at yourself. Are there ways you ask others to live as you want to live? What do you want to do about it?

A LIFE OF VALUE

One's life has value so long as one attributes value to the life of others, by means of love, friendship, indignation and compassion.

SIMONE DE BEAUVOIR

How do we value others' lives?

We listen to them. When we disagree with them, we try to see their point of view. No matter what they are saying, we look for a grain of truth in it. We become more interested in understanding them than in having them understand us.

We love them. We let ourselves explore intimacy by sharing ourselves and by listening to their sharing. We risk the vulnerability of love. We see them as both unique and like us, and we value both aspects. We honor the process of their lives, even though we may not always understand it.

We are a friend to them. We feel indignation when they are abused and offer support when it's needed. We are loyal without being blind. We are confrontational when necessary without being judgmental. We love them, and we let them know it.

We are compassionate. The humility of knowing that we don't run things and don't know it all undergirds compassion. Compassion is *feeling with* and *acting for.*

Study the above and see where it all fits in your life.

SELF-CENTEREDNESS

I used to believe that being self-centered was necessary for survival. Now I see it's killing me.

NORMA

When we are self-centered and self-seeking, we are so focused on ourselves—and yet so out of touch with ourselves—that we have difficulty letting anyone or anything else in. Our self-centeredness is an invisible wall that keeps us from ourselves even as it keeps others at bay. We become so absorbed in trying to manipulate people and circumstances to get what we need that we would not be able to see what we *really* need if it hit us over the head.

One cannot get out of self-centeredness through self-will. It just does not work. There are, however, two time-tested ways to deal with self-centeredness. The first is to do things for others, to be of service. Even if at first we may be doing service for *ourselves* in hope that we will feel better and the process eventually will work its magic.

The second is to return to that force of power that is greater than ourselves and hand our will and our lives over to it—and wait.

Self-centeredness is deadly to ourselves and to others. It's not worth what it costs us.

Try doing something of service today, just something simple for someone else. Don't tell anyone about it.

COOPERATION

The day of the dinosaurs is over. The future belongs to the bridge-builders, not the wreckers.

MARY MCALEESE

Rugged individualism is much easier than cooperation—or so we think. Tearing down is much easier than building—or so we think. Have we come to a time when the skills of the past are relegated to the past?

So many of us busy people have adopted an ethic of individual hard work, believing that this will get us what we want. We are willing to give a nod to team-building and cooperation, and down deep we still believe in the romanticism of the individual prevailing against all odds.

We have many tools to achieve on our own, yet, what do we know about participating in a work or living community? Even when we participate, are we able to know our self-hood and offer cooperation with the others? Is our time spent on power games? Are our coalitions really calculated moves? What do we know about "working with"?

List the skills you have to foster cooperation.

IMAGINATION AND HUMOR

Imagination was given to us to compensate for what we are not; a sense of humor was provided to console us for what we are.

MACK MCGINNIS

How precious are imagination and humor! What genius to put them together!

We need our imaginations to dream what can be and what we can become. Our imaginations allow us to soar beyond our physical limitations to places and worlds we might never have otherwise known. Our imaginations add to our stature and free our minds and souls for full flight. They add color, texture, dimension, energy, and magic to a world we might otherwise see as flat and colorless.

Our humor opens the door for us to gain perspective on ourselves and our human condition. Humor helps us see how ridiculous we are about the way we think things should be, and it lessens our tendency to trudge through life when we could skip. Humor is our reality check, urging us to take the serious lightly. Humor is our vehicle for insight—with a cherry on top. Humor is the salt of perspective in an otherwise unseasoned life.

Imagination and humor lift us out of the mud so that we can see what is possible in the stars.

Let your imagination lift you to what you can be while your humor keeps you from becoming too serious about what you are. Cultivate both traits in yourself.

THE HEALING POWER OF THE EARTH

One way to get expanded into a larger awareness of knowing and being is to "sit in the lap of Mother Earth" humbly with an Indian-friend, look off into scenic loveliness and far distances, and listen for the good counsel from the silence as it gently speaks to each of us in the infinite language of all life.

J. ALLEN BOONE

Native people the world over say that their myths and legends have told them that a time would come when their wisdom and knowledge would be needed to save the planet—that time is now. They are speaking out and making themselves available as never before.

Not all of us have native friends to call upon, and we do have the opportunity to return to the lap of our Mother, the earth, and hear the counsel of the silence.

My uncle, a Standing Rock Sioux, once told me, "When you are troubled, return to your Mother, the earth, press your face against her breast, and you will be healed." I have found this to be true. Just lying on the earth (without padding) does something for us. Everyone can do that.

When you feel confused, as if you have lost your way, go lie on your Mother, place your face on her breast, and listen to the "infinite language of all life."

INDIFFERENCE

The worst sin toward our fellow creatures is not to hate them, but to be indifferent to them; that's the essence of inhumanity.
GEORGE BERNARD SHAW

Where on earth did we get the idea that we have to be indifferent in order to survive? Somehow we have conceived the illusion that noticing and becoming involved in what is going on around us will be too much of a drain or more than we can handle. In the process, we have tried to "zombie-ize" ourselves and move carefully through the world in a protective shield of indifference.

Indifference is inhumane to others, and that's not the worst of it. It is absolutely devastating to ourselves. No wonder we feel off-balance. We *are.* We cannot be in balance unless we can feel with others. We fear both our feelings and the feelings of others. Yet, it is only through those feelings—ours *and* theirs— that we connect and return to wholeness.

It's not that we can't handle the feelings we have when we move through indifference to connectedness. We just need practice.

At home and/or at work, notice times of indifference. Practice being there for someone else, either by volunteering for something like AIDS *work or an agency such as the Humane Society. Or just let yourself feel when you watch the news on* TV.

DON'T SWEAT IT

There are two rules for living in harmony.
  1. Don't sweat the small stuff.
  2. It's all small stuff.

WAYNE DYER

Wayne Dyer wrote these words to Richard Carlson, who then used them as a title for his runaway best-selling book.

Learning not to grapple with every little thing that comes along is quite a struggle for many of us. The eggs are too runny; the coffee is not hot enough; the clothes don't fit exactly perfectly. Some of us have so fashioned our lives around perfecting the details of the small stuff that we never catch a glimpse of the bigger picture. We so distract our lives with details and convincing ourselves that *everything* matters that we live out of harmony and out of balance.

Everything is small stuff—that's a tougher one. Surely *some* things are not small stuff. Some of our issues, conflicts, and concerns are earth-shattering, or so they seem. What about the environment, our children, our retirement? Aren't these important? Perhaps. *And*, are they important enough to "sweat," and does sweating them make any difference?

The Serenity Prayer seems appropriate here:

God, grant me the serenity to accept the things I cannot change, the courage to change the things I can, and the wisdom to know the difference.

It's helpful to start each day with the Serenity Prayer. Say it more than once a day when needed.

CONTEXT, PARTICIPATION, CARING, AND RESPONSIBILITY

Always leave any place you go better than when you came to it.
VIRGIL WILLEY

This was a saying I heard my father repeat many times when I was growing up. Now, as an adult, I realize that it had a great influence upon me.

In saying this, my father was teaching me about context, participation, caring, and responsibility, all of which have served me well.

We live in *context.* When we know that we live in context and are part of a whole much bigger than ourselves, our self-centeredness disappears. We do not *use* people, places, or things, because they are part of and connected with us. When we went camping in my childhood, we picked up trash and other people's messes and left each place better than when we had arrived.

We need to *participate.* When I am passive in my life, I am out of balance. I am an onlooker. Picking up trash gave me the opportunity to be a participant. What a gift.

Through that gift I learned *caring.* As I cared for the campground, it became a part of me. I saw its beauty and wanted to help keep it beautiful.

I am *responsible.* I am responsible for what I do and what I don't do. No one else is. Complaining about those who had left trash didn't remove the trash. Picking it up did. I felt good about what *I* did and learned not to focus on what *they* did.

As you move through your day, check out context, participation, caring, and responsibility and see what these four concepts can contribute to your life.

THE LONELINESS OF WITHDRAWAL

Loneliness is never more cruel than when it is felt in close propinquity with someone who has ceased to communicate.

GERMAINE GREER

Most of us have been on both ends of this unsettling experience during our lives. When someone we know and love has drawn completely within themselves, the experience is that of being in a cold, dark, damp cave with no stimulation or warmth coming from any direction. We find ourselves in a situation of sensory deprivation. In this state, our self-esteem plummets, and we feel grateful for the butcher or anyone else who greets us as if he likes us. Perceptions become distorted, and miasma sets in.

When we withdraw like this ourselves, it is equally devastating to those around us. When my daughter was two years old, I came home from the doctor's office with news of a questionable Pap smear. I was frightened and drew into myself. My daughter could sense my fear immediately and she refused to let me withdraw into my frightened self. I was in such a state of shock that I did not think of the effect my withdrawal would have on her. And, she did! She picked away at my wall relentlessly until I had to let her in. I was grateful.

When someone withdraws from you and won't let you in, make sure you spend time with others who love you and will listen to you. Remember that you have yourself as well.

When you withdraw, be aware of the destructive effect it has on others. Force yourself to talk to those who care for you.

HIDING OUR POWER

She posed as being more indolent than she felt, for fear of finding herself less able than she could wish.

ELIZABETH BOWEN

How often we stop ourselves before we start, fearing our own possible inadequacy. We are so afraid of not having the right skills or knowledge (and that others, God forbid, will see it) that we spend much of our time trying to make ourselves look much less adequate than we are. What if we fail?

Also, appearing inadequate is a kind of safety net. People don't like adequate people, we rationalize, so why set ourselves up? If we prove ourselves to be more adequate than we or they believe we are, they may expect more from us—then we'd really be in trouble! No telling who would go after us if they knew how good we are. Plus, our secret powers give us an edge over others—don't they?

What deadly games we play with ourselves! We avoid the risk of making a mistake even though mistakes are one of our greatest forms of learning. We hide our power and then wonder why we feel powerless. We give others the position to determine what we know and don't know and then resent them for having power over us. No wonder we feel off-balance!

Quit playing games with yourself and others. Let yourself and those you associate with see how good you are. Come out of your closet as a knowledgeable person. So you make a few mistakes—so what? Use them as springboards for learning.

GRATITUDE

Sometimes we need to remind ourselves that thankfulness is indeed virtue.

WILLIAM J. BENNETT

I recently had an experience that resulted in my looking at gratitude from a totally different perspective. I had been traveling and working for several months. I had taken good care of myself, and I still felt tired and a little off-balance (it may be age). My son also felt burnt out, so I suggested that we both go to a spa for a couple of days. It was just what we needed. At the spa, my feet were rubbed and massaged many times.

Now, my feet have not been too happy of late. A few years ago I had an accident: my left foot was almost cut off by a machete. Since then, pain in that foot has been an almost constant companion. On my right foot, the joint of my big toe has had two sieges of excruciating goutlike pain. At the spa, I was aware of the absence of pain in my feet and of how good that felt. I could have foot rubs and massages and *no pain.*

I suddenly realized how grateful I was for the absence of pain in my feet. Then I started ticking off other absences for which I was grateful—the absence of certain very difficult people in my life, the absence of feelings of resentment toward those who have "wronged" me, the absence of feelings of loss for relationships and things long gone—and on and on. We have such a range of gratitude possibilities. I could see how far I had come.

Make a gratitude list of the absences for which you are grateful. See how much you have done and how far you have come. Add to it regularly.

HOUSEWORK

I think housework is the reason most women go to the office.
HELOISE

Ah, housework! What book about balance would be complete without a look at housework? When we hear that death and taxes are the only things that are inevitable, housework also comes to mind. Regardless of the kind of home we have set up for ourselves, regardless of the busy, important worklife we have carved out, regardless of the kinds of arrangements we have concocted to avoid it—wives, househusbands, housekeepers, quiet ignoring—there housework is, silently and surely confronting us with its reproaching gaze.

Quentin Crisp once said something like this: "After a few years the dirt doesn't get any deeper, so forget it." I tried that and discovered that in fact it *does*. Dust gets *deeper*—can you believe it? Dust may be the one thing in our lives that is proven to be limitless. We look for limitlessness in love, in money, in power, in prestige—and we find it in dust. What a hoot!

Maybe our main difficulty with housework is ourselves.

Let yourself laugh about your struggle with housework. Then, maybe you will have the opportunity to take it one step at a time and enjoy it.

Approach dusting and vacuuming as a moving meditation and see if anything changes.

SELF-RELIANCE

We cannot climb up a rope that is attached only to our own belt.
WILLIAM ERNEST HOCKING

Rarely do we take the time to examine the philosophies that guide or confine our day-to-day living. So subtle is the influence of some of these philosophies that we do not even have a conscious awareness of their existence. Take self-reliance for example.

Self-reliance is part of the warp and woof of the American culture; it is an ideal that permeates much of how and what we think and feel. Yet, self-reliance is a difficult issue for many of us. Self-reliance has been twisted to mean that we have to do everything for ourselves, that asking for help is an act of losing face. In our culture, heroes are people who never need anyone else (and even when they accept help, they don't really need it).

Perhaps most of us would stop right there and loudly decry, "This is too extreme for me. It doesn't apply."

Doesn't it? Take a closer look.

Do we secretly feel like failures when we don't know how to do everything ourselves? Do we push ourselves beyond our comfort level and beyond our level of expertise? Have we "given up" because we unconsciously hold on to a belief in self-reliance but just can't do it all? Are we so self-sufficient that we don't know how to function cooperatively?

A balanced life invites us to learn to take responsibility and use our talents, and yet it also reminds us that a rope held by many hands is stronger than a rope held by only one.

Check out your beliefs, illusions, and philosophies about self-reliance.

CHILD-REARING

The reason for the success of Clan of the Cave Bear *is that it's about a Cro-Magnon child being raised by a family of Neanderthals—a position almost all of us have been in.*

LAWRENCE BLOCK

Current psychological theory tells us that we can be scarred for life by our parents. That's one theory, and it certainly gets us off the hook. Let's take another perspective and see where it gets us. What if we drop our perfect family and *Leave It to Beaver* illusions, instead viewing the family we were born into as the raw material we were given for learning the lessons we need in life. Not all raw material looks good at first and the secret is not in the material; the secret is in what we do with it.

Our families and our childhoods are our realities. When viewed from this perspective, it is possible to see the experiences as neither good or bad—they just are. It's what we do with them that makes them what they are. We have the opportunity to glean some gems of learning from what may have been very painful or very happy situations. If we choose only to hold on to past hurts, we die with them. Transformation is in our hands.

Are there issues from childhood you use as a crutch to avoid running with life? Check this out.

WONDER

There are no seven wonders of the world in the eyes of a child. There are seven million.

WALT STREIGHTIFF

Never lose the ability to experience wonder. Wonder is one of the greatest balancers we possess.

Several years ago, I went through a period of feeling at sixes and sevens. Nothing was really wrong, and yet nothing was really right either. I felt off-balance—tilted and uneasy. I tried *thinking* myself out of this state. I did good and bad lists, right and wrong lists, and action lists. I even squeezed in a couple of affirmations. Nothing worked. I trusted that this state would not continue forever, and I sure didn't like it much. In true human style, I felt I should do something about it. I was willing to tackle it, and I was at a loss as to what might work.

In desperation, I walked out in the yard one night and looked up. The stars were out, and some were shooting across the sky. Without consciously forcing it, the wonder I felt returned me to balance, and I walked back into the house at peace.

Sometimes we can't *bring* our lives back into balance. We have to *allow* them to return to balance.

"Allowing" our lives to flow is one of the wonders of life. Try "allowing" with wonder.

CHILDREN—LEARNING

A child becomes an adult when he realizes he has a right not only to be right but also to be wrong.

THOMAS SZASZ

The most important right a child has is to be a child. A child is not an immature or incomplete adult. A child is a child.

One of the most exciting aspects about childhood is that it is a time when accelerated learning is not only possible; it is expected and supported by society. It's probably not that children are capable of more or faster learning than adults. We have all just agreed that childhood is a time when learning is desirable.

We can all learn as much and as fast as children throughout our lives. In fact, I've concluded that, contrary to popular opinion, children tend to be more rigid than adults and therefore sometimes have a more difficult time learning. If we didn't push our children to become little adults, they probably would not be as inclined to respond with rigidity.

When we give ourselves the right to be right and the right to be wrong, we are neither children nor adults; we are human beings.

See yourself as being as capable as a child is of great gobs of learning. Start by learning something you have always wanted to learn.

LONELINESS

Loneliness is often the missing of ourselves.

ANNE

Loneliness is one of the most feared states in modern life. Perhaps this fear has come about because so many of us have a vague awareness of a surging river of loneliness deep inside. Much of our activity and busyness is designed to keep that river within its banks.

Maybe loneliness has received a bad rap in today's world. Maybe loneliness is one of the ways our inner being communicates with us, letting us know that we need to take the time to get back in touch with ourselves. Could it be that the emptiness we feel in our solar plexus (and try so hard to avoid) is a friendly reminder that something (or someone!) has gone missing—we *ourselves!*

Try as we might, we can never fill up this void with anything outside ourselves—any person, activity, or thing. We can wear ourselves out *trying* to fill up this hole, but this approach alleviates the feeling for only a short while. Eventually we have to get back to ourselves. We are, after all, why we're here.

When we are lonely, it's usually a signal that we need to spend some time with ourselves. The next time you get this signal, try taking some time alone.

PRAYER

It doesn't matter what things you pray for—it's always better to pray for people.

SUSAN

Have you tried praying lately?

In many circles, praying is a bit out of style; it's done only in extreme circumstances of life and death. In other circles, praying has become a meaningless mumbo-jumbo of mindless ritual, full of words with little heart.

Some say that the simplest prayers—such as a single word, *Help!*—are best. Others believe that we have to be taught to pray and that certain rituals and procedures work best. Still others are so frightened off by all this that they don't go near prayer.

My experience is that no one has a corner on prayer. There are as many ways to pray as there are living beings on this planet. Some say that we can live our life as a prayer, every act and deed goes beyond ourselves into that vast mystery that is greater than ourselves. Perhaps the trees have perfected prayer as they steadfastly lift their branches skyward.

What I do know is that one of the most effective prayers is a prayer for someone who has wronged you. When we can do this without piety and with sincerity and compassion, we can truly learn the lessons that this experience has to teach us and bring our lives back into balance.

Try praying for someone who has wronged you. Sincerely!

FRIENDSHIP

No person is your friend who demands your silence, or denies your right to grow.

ALICE WALKER

Friendship is so precious—and so necessary. We need friends to serve as mirrors so that we can see ourselves. A good friend clearly sees our faults, reflects them back to us, and loves us through them.

When we are insecure in ourselves and reluctant to grow and change, we will choose friends who support our stasis, agree with all our opinions, and demand our silence. When we see our friends acting this way, we must remember that we have chosen them. We reveal a lot about ourselves in the friends we choose.

Our good friends may not always agree with us, yet they never demand our silence when our perspectives differ. Good friends rejoice in our right to grow and in our growth, even if that means that we grow away from them. We are a good friend to others when we do the same thing.

Friendship is not a vehicle for control; it is a vehicle for freedom. It is a system that is open in all directions for those who participate.

Take a look at what kinds of friends you are choosing and what kind of friend you are.

HEALTH

Indians . . . know better how to live . . . Nobody can be in good health if he does not have all the time fresh air, sunshine, and good water.

CHIEF FLYING HAWK

For most of us, good health is a choice and, for all of us, it is a choice within our limitations. There was a time in the history of our nation, and of the world, that fresh air, sunshine, and good water were givens; they were understood as rights for us all. That time no longer exists. We have become so accustomed to the pollution of our food, air, and water that we just passively accept contamination as our reality. This passive acceptance of harmful elements need not continue. It's up to each and every one of us to move into the deep knowing that we do not *have* to live like this.

We will not restore the balance of fresh air, sunshine, and good water unless all of us know that these elements are our rights, and we deserve them. Only when we as individuals rank a healthy environment as a priority in our lives will things change. Only when we become dedicated to our children's future and the future of six generations after them will we see ourselves as part of a greater whole.

Look around your home and find at least three ways to make your living environment more healthy—more living plants, fewer toxic cleaning products, healthier food, cleaner water, and more supportive friendships. Then do something about improving the situation.

DELVING DEEP

When you understand one thing through and through, you understand everything.

SHUNRYU SUZUKI

There's just too much—too much to learn, too much to see, too much to do, too much information, too much technology, too many techniques, too many ways to pleasure, too many ways to pain. Too much!

How can we be expected to take it all in and deal with it?

Perhaps we don't have to take it all in *or* deal with it.

What a relief to know that we can go deeper and deeper into whatever we wish, and through that exploration come to understand the everything. Since all of creation is a whole and the oneness of all creation is a reality, our world is indeed a holomovement or hologram. In exploring the depths of one thing, we gain wisdom about others. Our task, then, is to see what calls to us, what piques our imagination, what stimulates our being and asks us to delve deeper and deeper into it. When we follow this calling, we will find balance.

Delve deeper into something that fascinates you. Uncover at least one piece of information that helps you know the subject better and jot it down.

EXPANDING OUR HORIZONS

Que será será
What will be will be.

This was one of my favorite songs when I was younger—
Good old Doris Day. The phrase *"Que será será"* became totally
integrated into the culture with that song, though most of us
didn't know we were speaking Spanish at that tender age. It was
a good song—no doubt about it—and it was more than that. It
became commonplace, I believe, because the wisdom of "What
will be will be" struck a chord we all needed to hear.

We are a world of so many cultures, so many approaches to
wisdom, so many varied ways of communicating truth, that it
seems out of balance not to open ourselves up to the myriad wis-
doms that are all around us.

When we read books only from our own particular culture
or religion, we rob ourselves of experiencing the richness that
diversity brings. What are we afraid of? Do we truly think that
our beliefs and wisdom can't stand up to other beliefs? Have we
deluded ourselves into thinking that our truths are the only
truths?

We need other wisdom and truths to bring balance to our
lives.

Go get a book from another culture or belief system—one
that will stretch you. Make opportunities to experience
something of other cultures other than their food.

VICES

It has been my experience that folks who have no vices have very few virtues.

ABRAHAM LINCOLN

What a relief! Vices are bad. Virtues are good. Everyone knows that. Yet what if there is another way to look at vices and virtues? Don't you just love it when there is another way to look at something that has been around for a long time?

What if our filtering mechanisms are not as sophisticated as we would like them to be? Many of us know that this tends to be true about feelings. It seems that we can't filter out just the "bad" feelings (anger, disgust, lust, misery, and stinginess) and let the "good" ones (love, joy, happiness, and caring) through. When we start filtering feelings, we filter *all* feelings, not *particular* feelings.

Maybe it is the same way with vices and virtues. When we try to hide or control our vices, we conceal and control our virtues as well.

Martin Luther said, "Sin bravely so that grace may abound."

Perhaps it is through coming to grips with our vices that we gain the humility to be virtuous.

Make a list of the vices you most hate to admit . Then list some of your greatest virtues. See what you can learn from these lists. Are you ready to give up some of the vices and admit to some of the virtues?

RESPONSIBILITY

There is a quiet, serene confidence in knowing that all things do not stand or fall according to one's own achievements or the correctness of every decision one makes.

JOSEPH A. SITTLER

One of the burdens that we people who do too much put on ourselves is feeling responsible for everything. Actually, one of our favorite dualisms—one on which we painfully dance—is that at one end we are responsible for everything, with the weight of the world resting on our shoulders, while at the other end, we want to chuck it all, head for the woods, and live in a cave. Like most dualisms, neither extreme seems too appealing. This dualism teeters on the fulcrum of self-centeredness.

When we realize that we are responsible for what we do and need to take ownership for our thoughts, actions, and behaviors and realize at the same time that we do not control everything, we can relax a bit.

We can do the best we can and then let go.

Are you too hard on yourself in a self-centered way? Can you do the best you can and let go?

Try the Serenity Prayer:

God, grant me the serenity to accept the things I cannot change, the courage to change the things I can, and the wisdom to know the difference.

ACTION

Manifestation is only given when action is taken.

MARICARDA

Those of us who do too much tend to see ourselves as people of action. This may be one of our favorite illusions. Could we possibly have confused *activity* with *action*? Just because we are in motion doesn't necessarily mean we are doing something. Procrastination, confusion, busywork, and avoidance may all involve activity, though nothing gets done as a result of them.

Things get done only when we actually *do* something. I can think about what I am going to fix for dinner for hours. I can plan elaborate menus. I can study recipes and set the table. All of these activities may expend large amounts of energy, and yet dinner isn't cooked. Bill Gates could have had a ton of great ideas, and unless he expedited them he would never have had millions to give away.

Planning, plotting, and pursuing ideas are great, and yet it is the focused action that brings results.

Busy people can run roughshod over action on their path of busyness.

Only our actions will lead us to what we want.

What actions do you need to take to manifest something you have been wanting?

A NEW DAY

Today is a new day. You will get out of it just what you put into it. If you have made mistakes, even serious mistakes, there is always another chance for you. And supposing you have tried and failed again and again, you may have a fresh start any moment you choose, for this thing that we call "failure" is not the falling down, but the staying down.

MARY PICKFORD

How exciting it is to approach each day as a new day, which of course, it is.

There is something about the freshness in the idea of a new day that encourages us to shake the dust off our sandals and give life a new try.

We can begin again each day. Each new day brings with it the opportunity to come up with fresh ideas, fresh approaches, and fresh behaviors.

This doesn't mean that we ignore the past or pretend that we do not have to deal with it. We do. And, when we approach each morning as a new day with new possibilities, our lives beckon us.

Greet each day as a new day rich with possibilities, and see what happens.

CHAOS

Before anything is brought back into order, it is quite normal for it to be brought first into a kind of confusion, a virtual chaos. In this way, things that fit together badly are severed from each other; and when they have been severed, then God arranges them in order.

EMANUEL SWEDENBORG

Swedenborg was one of the early chaos theorists.

If we really want balance in our lives, we need to be able to accept, tolerate, and even embrace chaos. All too often, we find ourselves trying to put together things that fit badly. Two woods that cure at different rates and in different ways, for example, don't do well when laminated together. And all too often we want to believe that love is enough to hold together two people who are headed in very different directions. Sometimes, out of self-will and stubbornness, we try to hold on to a job that we know deep down we don't even like or maybe aren't good at.

We refuse the severing and the resulting chaos and as a consequence miss the possible resultant order that "God arranges."

When we learn to see chaos as a precursor of order, we are making progress.

When chaos prevails, see if you can see it as a movement toward balance.

WORK

Work is not, primarily, a thing one does to live, but the thing one lives to do. It is, or it should be, the full expression of the worker's faculties.

DOROTHY SAYERS

Work and love are not opposites. When we love our work, we experience great balance. One of the ways we can bring love and balance to our work is to let ourselves recognize the gift we have been given in doing it.

Work is sacred. It is not just a way to earn money or gain power, though it may result in both.

Work is a vehicle for testing out our gifts and talents and using them to explore their meaning. Work is a process of self-expression, trial-and-error learning, creativity, and risk-taking. No matter what kind of job we have, work always has these potentials.

Work is spiritual. It is a place where we have the opportunity for spiritual growth. Often these opportunities come from the "how" of the ways we do our work rather than the "what" of the work itself.

Regardless of what our work is, we can enjoy it. And it is most enjoyable when balanced with other aspects of our life and not a tyrant.

How do you approach your work? Are there some things you need to modify?

FEELING CRAZY

That's the truest sign of insanity—insane people are always sure they're just fine. It's only the sane people who are willing to admit they're crazy.

NORA EPHRON

Feeling crazy may be a mark of sanity, a sign that our reality testing is effective.

Most of us come from dysfunctional families (though they may have looked like *The Brady Bunch*), since dysfunctional families are the norm for today's society. During our early years we learned valuable skills for functioning in dysfunction, skills that we have carried into our adulthood.

We go to workplaces that can be quite insane at times, and yet when we name the insanity, we're told we're crazy.

We see our leaders say one thing and do another. We can't listen to a political speech without all of our con-detector bells going off.

We want our relationships to function—no, thrive—and we have very few models of healthy relating.

Feeling crazy may be a normal response to crazy situations. It may be a form of balancing.

The next time you feel a bit crazy, honor the feeling and be open to the possibility that feeling crazy might be a normal response in that situation.

IMAGE MANAGEMENT

*The art of never making a mistake is crucial to motherhood.
To be effective and to gain the respect she needs to function, a
mother must have her children believe she has never engaged in sex,
never made a bad decision, never caused her own mother a moment's
anxiety, and was never a child.*

ERMA BOMBECK

The wonderful thing about good humor is that it always
reveals with piercing truthfulness some of our cherished illusions that we are usually not ready to abandon. Image control is
one of our favorites.

We like to justify our subtle image management under the
guise that we need people to see us a certain way in order for us
to do our job. Ministers need to be seen as holy, teachers as
knowledgeable, and parents as perfect.

At some point, however, we need to ask ourselves, "Is a *role*
raising our children? Is a *myth* guiding our spiritual progress? Is
a *robot* teaching our children?"

When we finally grasp the reality that our very humanness
is what makes us shine and that our impression management is
for naught, humility sets in and we can give what we have.

*Are there areas in your life in which you typically engage in
image management? How do you feel about it? Is it worth
it? Could you be more yourself and still get the job done?
What's important to you?*

UNFAIRNESS

It takes six months to get into shape and two weeks to get out of shape. Once you know this you can stop being angry about other things in life and only be angry about this.

RITA RUDNER

What a great idea—an impersonal focus for our anger and rage.

It's even better if we expand the picture a little bit to get a broader perspective, accepting that in general life isn't fair.

Way back when I was younger I spent a lot of time exclaiming that it (whatever "it" was!) wasn't fair. Whenever I saw something that I perceived as being unfair (and, of course, there were examples all around me), I became indignant, self-righteous, infuriated, and sometimes (very rarely, of course) combative. As I look back, I'm not sure that any of these reactions accomplished much except to get me exhausted, beat-up, resentful, and in trouble.

It took me a long time to come to the realization that life isn't fair. That's my reality and everyone else's. I don't have to like it. I *do* have to accept it. Life just isn't fair. I can't possibly see the whole picture, and, from my limited view, life isn't fair.

Once the conclusion has been accepted, how do I move on? I can be as fair as I can, given my limitations. I can accept reality and move on. I can be kind, considerate, caring, patient, and supportive in dealing with those who experience great unfairness.

Do you fight the unfairness of life? You could accept it and move on, contributing what you can.

ACHIEVEMENT

Somewhere I learned that I had to be tough, driven, and pushy to get anything done. I have no idea where I got that.

STANLEY

Where do we get these ideas? We bend ourselves and others around us like pretzels because somewhere we were told that only those who are driven succeed. We fear that if we are caring and peaceful, others will take advantage of us, see us as push-overs, and we won't achieve anything.

There are those who try to take advantage of anyone or any-thing they see as soft or gentle and those are probably the same people who will also try to take advantage of people they see as tough.

The real issue is what is happening to us in the process. Do we like ourselves when we are tough, driven, and pushy?

We can be strong without being tough. We can be produc-tive without being driven. We can stand up for ourselves with-out being pushy.

Gentle, loving, peaceful people *do* get a lot done. They are achievers—who like themselves.

See how you can change driven into productive, holding your ground *for being* pushy, *being* strong *for being* tough—*being* balanced *for being* off-balance.

SMILING

A smile is the universal welcome.

MAX EASTMAN

There is an old Irish saying that goes something like this: "There are no strangers here, just friends we haven't met yet."

Openness and friendliness are two of the best investments we can make. They consistently yield very high dividends.

There is a belief that it is unsophisticated to be too open and friendly; that people might even take advantage of us if we smile at them. Avoiding eye contact and not smiling at strangers has become the norm, feeding our escape from intimacy with others and with ourselves.

Rumor has it that it takes seventeen muscles to smile and forty-three muscles to frown. Smiling is a lot less work. In addition, we tend to feel good about ourselves when we smile and offer a friendly hello to those we meet.

I have noticed that whenever I see a child, my face and being want to smile. When I do, the child almost always focuses on me. Because I have initiated a smile for that child, we share a moment of love and intimacy. What could possibly be better than that?

Try offering smiles to those you meet. You'll like how you feel. Don't look down; make eye contact.

INTERRUPTING OTHERS

One of the things I do when I get too busy is that I interrupt people when they are talking.

SUEANN

When we were children, most of us were taught that it was rude to interrupt others when they were speaking. We were taught to listen and wait until the speaker had finished before we spoke.

As we became busy adults, we grew too rushed and too "important" to observe this suggestion for sane living.

Once in a while, it is good to stop long enough to check out some of the basics we were taught as a child, testing their relevance for our lives today.

When we interrupt other people, we are often more concerned with what *we* have to say than with what *they* have to say. Is this a message we want to send? When we interrupt, we may be trying to speed things along, make them go faster so that we can get on to other things, or just rush in general. We become so addicted to rushing on to the next thing, and then the *next* thing becomes what we want to rush away from, and so it goes.

Our interrupting others may be one of the lovely red flags, warning us of the need to stop to notice what we are doing to ourselves and others.

Notice your tendency to interrupt, and deliberately allow others to finish what they are saying. Notice how this seems to reduce tension.

ADVICE

Get the advice of everybody whose advice is worth having—they are very few—and then do what you think best yourself.

CHARLES STEWART PARNELL

Advice is tricky. We usually seek it only when we do not want to take responsibility for our own decisions, when we do not want to make a decision, or when we want to reject it. Rarely do we approach advice-gathering honestly.

In order to gather advice honestly, we have to feel strong enough in ourselves to be genuinely open to what is said, being open to changing our previous opinion. Many people believe they can do this; few can. Second, we have to be in a position clearly to weigh the information shared to see what is valuable for us. Then, we have to be able and willing to move forward with our decision, knowing that it is *our* decision and that we are responsible for it regardless of the advice given.

Getting advice can be very valuable if we understand how to use it.

Don't give advice to those who don't know how to use it, and don't ask for advice if you can't use it judiciously.

SELF-IMPROVEMENT

There is only one way in which it [healing the planet] can be done, and that is by individual purification and refinement. As each of us improves himself, he helps the world just that much. As he neglects to improve himself, he holds the world back just that much.

ANONYMOUS (QUOTED BY J. ALLEN BOONE)

Our personal work—what we do to grow and evolve—does make a difference. Time and time again I have seen brilliant people with powerful messages undo themselves (and their message) because they have refused to do their own personal work. They negate the impact they might have had by setting themselves above others and refusing to admit that they, too, are here to evolve and work on their spiritual journeys.

We all have such a marvelous opportunity in this life to evolve, grow, and move more and more toward becoming all we can be. At the end of our lives, who we are and what that has contributed to the process of healing the planet will probably be much more important than anything we have produced or done for money, fame, or power.

We are a piece of the puzzle of the universe. Taking our place as the fullest piece we can be will probably be our most precious contribution.

Have you lost your way? Is your spiritual path front and center with you? Do you need to reevaluate what's important to you?

TAKING THINGS
AS THEY COME

It is far better to take things as they come along with patience and equanimity.

CARL JUNG

I recently set out to make contact with a rather well known writer in Ireland. I thought that I knew where he lived and it would be easy to find him. My first afternoon yielded nothing. I couldn't find the road, the village, or the house. I decided to make one last try on the way to the airport. My first foray up an unmarked mountain road yielded (1) an interesting man who had just moved in and knew none of the neighbors; (2) a discovery of a "village" I didn't know existed; (3) a beautiful drive and view; and (4) an old-timer who knew *approximately* where the writer lived and gave me *almost* right directions.

Deciding that we were hot on the trail, we agreed to forgo our dinner reservations at a restaurant that came highly recommended. We ended up at a fish factory, where I closed my finger in the door (very painful). Workers there pointed us in the right direction. After three false turns, discovering another village we didn't know existed, and visiting with two lovely Gaelic-speaking families, we found our writer. He had just driven up to his house from a trip overseas. If we had found the house on the first try, he would not have been there.

Practice taking things as they come with patience and equanimity. Don't fight life.

BODYCARE

The body is a sacred garment.

MARTHA GRAHAM

There are times when we simply need to care for our bodies. We need to learn to act before they are screaming for attention; we should do some routine maintenance care as we go along. It makes it possible to stay in them as we move through life, even when the going gets rough. Caring for our bodies is one of the major ways we can return to balance.

One of the most effective ways we can care for our bodies is to give ourselves an at-home spa treatment. Periodically we need to let go of old, worn-out, useless parts of ourselves. Nothing feels better than ridding ourselves of old, dead skin.

Start with coarse sea salt (preferably Hawaiian) in a thick cream or lotion. Gently rub it all over your body, giving yourself a good scrub. (It's really nice if you can do this with someone else.) Fill the bathroom with steam and sit for a while, letting the sea salt and lotion "melt" and soak in. The sea salt replenishes ninety-seven trace minerals and elements that get depleted as we go through life. After sitting for a while, get in a nice warm shower and scrub off the sea salt and lotion with a loofah. Before drying, pumice your feet and any other rough spots on the body—elbows, knees, ankles. Then dry off, cream or oil yourself with lavender or a fragrance that is calming, and rest.

You'll be glad you took the time, and your body will give you positive feedback.

RANDOM KINDNESS,
SENSELESS BEAUTY

Practice random acts of kindness and senseless acts of beauty.
ANONYMOUS BUMPER STICKER

This bumper sticker appeared all over the country a few years ago, grabbing the imagination of everyone who saw it.

What joy we find in random acts of kindness. (Premeditated acts of kindness are fine too.) They add a certain spring to our step. The randomness seems to transmute the kindness, adding a spontaneity that surprises even the doer. There is something playful about being spontaneous with our kindness that restores the innocence of childhood and the fun of being young. Whatever the chemistry of random acts of kindness, we benefit immeasurably from them.

Senseless acts of beauty have the same restorative power. It is easy to become so routinized and sensible in our creation of beauty. Our gardens become "organized," the art in our houses become stylized, and our clothes are coordinated. What a release it is to practice *senseless* acts of beauty. One has the feeling of flying just from reading the words. I planted a cypress tree where it really doesn't "belong." It's so beautiful!

Open yourself to random acts of kindness and senseless acts of beauty. I won't make suggestions—that would destroy the randomness. You can do it. Keep your eyes and ears open for possibilities.

WORRY

When you borrow trouble you give your peace of mind as security.
MYRTLE REED

Why in the world would we borrow trouble when there are so many more interesting things we could borrow? Yet we *do* borrow trouble when we worry. Worry is one of the most debilitating and unbalancing activities of human existence.

Those of us who are worriers know that once initiated, worry takes on a life of its own. It is like one of those self-relighting gas heaters that just goes on and on. Or, to use a more ominous image, worry is like quicksand, sucking us under once we stick our toes in. Worry is one area where expertise is not celebrated and those who are good at it find no enjoyment.

Most people don't realize that worry is a form of control. When we worry, we are trying to control an outcome. We have made our worrying a necessary part of the equation. Unfortunately, there is nothing so self-defeating and unbalancing as trying to control something over which we have no control.

When you start to worry over something, stop to realize that you have no control and see what positive action you can take.

SKILLS FOR LIVING

If logic tells you that life is a meaningless accident, don't give up on life. Give up on logic.

SHIRA MILGROM

There's nothing wrong with logic. Logic is a wonderful thing. It is so reasonable, so accurate, and so rational when we are dealing with issues that are reasonable, rational, and logical. It's also useful when we are focusing on conceptualizations on the material plane of life. Technology, mechanics, and logic all have their place. They also, however, have their limitations.

No matter what thinking processes (or other tools) we are using, we will be more balanced if we are clear about when they are useful and when they are not. We need to use them only when it is appropriate. This, of course, means we need to develop a wide range of abilities and responses within ourselves and know how to use them.

For example, logic is next to useless when it comes to understanding life. Life is best understood with feelings, intuition, and awareness. These processes are just as wise as logic. They just cover a different territory.

When we try to use skills that don't apply in one area of our life and ignore the development of other, necessary skills, we suffer; we get out of balance; we tilt. When we have a range of skills and are willing to use them appropriately, life proceeds—and much more easily.

Take a look at your thinking and perceiving skills and see which need work.

INTIMACY

The only thing worth stealing is a kiss from a sleeping child.
JOE HOULDSWORTH

What an intimate experience it is to watch someone you love sleeping! Whether the loved one is a pet, a baby, or a partner, the intimacy that emanates from the quietness and vulnerability cannot be experienced in any other way. How open and peaceful our loved ones are when they are sleeping. They are not having to relate to us, notice us, or focus on us. Their defenses are down, and they exude a vulnerability that may not be there at any other time.

There are so many ways we escape from intimacy that we need to take every opportunity, learn every possible way, to let intimacy in.

At a spa I enjoy, I recently witnessed what I perceived to be an escape from intimacy. I had heard a young woman say that she and her boyfriend had come to the spa because he was exhausted. He had just had a massage, sat down in an easy chair, and immediately fell asleep. He looked wonderfully peaceful. She buzzed into the room and did not skip a beat in waking him up. I felt sad as I watched an intimacy missed. I also felt grateful for the reminder to "wait with" those intimate moments—whatever and wherever they are.

Look at the subtle, tiny ways you escape from intimacy. Is that avoidance what you really want?

QUARRELS

Quarrels in France strengthen a love affair, in America they end it.
NED ROREM

How much fun it is to fight and then kiss and make up! Yet, the fight may not be the real issue here. So many fights are not about the seeming focus of the fight. Fights are often a vehicle for something else. Ultimately, fights are usually about two issues: intimacy and needing space.

Intimacy is a big issue in our lives. Most of us are convinced that we are desperate for intimacy and actively go after it; and yet we typically seek intimacy in ways that are sure to prevent it, such as sex, romance, adrenaline, or physical attraction. These approaches are undergirded by a deep fear of intimacy and a need to control the emotional distance we have with others. If we are not intimate with ourselves, how can we be intimate with anyone else?

Another major reason we fight is because we need some alone time—time and space for ourselves—and we don't know how to take it gracefully. Therefore, we effectively drive the other person away. We then assure ourselves that he or she went by choice so that we don't have to take responsibility for the alone time we need. Tricky and effective and, is this really what we want?

The next time a quarrel is brewing, check out the issues of intimacy, alone time, and control within yourself.

SLEEP

I love to sleep! It is one of my better skills.

ELIZABETH

Busy people think of sleep as a waste of time or as an objectionable necessity that interferes with the *real* meaning of life: getting things done.

Sleep is absolutely essential as a means by which we rest and refurbish our bodies. And it is certainly much, much more.

Sleep is a magical process that transports us into other realms, into other times and places. In sleep, time and space have no meaning. We can be in any time, in any space. Sleep is a state in which we solve problems, work through unfinished, deep processes, and attend classes in the inner university of self and universe.

Have you ever tried to share the intricacies of a dream with someone or even write it down for yourself? If so, you no doubt experienced how woefully inadequate the rational mind is at describing a dream. You can *see* the dream in your mind. Yet, words fail to capture the richness of the experience. It is not only the body that regenerates during sleep, the mind and soul also heal and grow.

Look at your attitude toward sleep. See if you need to change it to be more balanced.

LIVING IN THE PRESENT

*The past has flown away. The coming month and year do not exist.
Ours only is the present's tiny point.*

MAHMUD SHABISTARI

Living in the present is like trying to balance on "the present's tiny point" in toe shoes. Falling into the future or the past is always a more-than-likely possibility.

In the past, when I heard beautiful words about living in the present, I would generally think, "Well, this living in the present is a beautiful sentiment, *and . . .* it's not really a practical reality." I would feel pleased with myself for valuing the sentiment of living in the present, and yet I would keep doing what I had been doing.

Then one day—I got it! I realized that living in the present is not an *idea*. It's *reality*. It's like taking one step at a time. Sounds good. Good philosophy, right? Then it occurred to me, Have you ever tried to take two steps at a time? We can't. It's as simple as that: we can't.

It's the same with living in the present. Our thoughts may wander to the past or the future. Yet, our thoughts are just thoughts. Our bodies are in the present. We are in the present. That's just the way it is.

Look around you. What is your present today? What steps can you take to live in it more fully?

OLD FRIENDS AND LOVERS

It's relaxing to go out with my ex-wife because she already knows I'm an idiot.

WARREN THOMAS

It's important to have people in our lives who are like old shoes. In this age of disposable everything, old husbands, lovers, wives, boyfriends, and girlfriends can offer a unique balance to our lives. Relationships change over time. This is the reality of relationships. If we are able to change with them, their continuation can add great richness to our lives.

People with whom we were once very close add a perspective to our lives that no one else can. (Likewise, we can add a perspective to their lives that no one else can.) If we are willing to do our own personal work—processing and letting go of old resentments and grievances—these people can be storehouses of memories and perceptions that can enrich us immeasurably. They and their current partners and spouses knew a person who may no longer be front and center and yet, is a part of the person we are now. The ability to laugh together over past rigidities and foibles can go a long way toward healing and balance.

As we grow, we may be able to see that the reason we needed to leave a former relationship was that the other person already knew we were being an idiot.

Are there people from your past you need to be friends with? What do you need to do about this?

A SEPARATE WORKSPACE

I have learned to keep my work separate from everything else.
RICHARD CARLSON

These days, when work seems to permeate every aspect of our lives and balance and efficiency have been sacrificed for the constancy of work, the suggestion that we separate work from the rest of our lives seems impossible. Yet, in that very impossibility lies the reason that such separation is even more necessary.

In the times of our great grandfathers, life and work were totally integrated and everyone pitched in on all levels. Now much of our work is done with our heads, and much of it is high-tech. Indeed, much of it requires that we be out of our bodies, as it were, and not really present.

Whether out of an office or in our home, we all need a workplace that is our own. We need a place where we can close the door and know that it will stay closed until we open it. We need a place where we can withdraw, giving us a chance fully to return. We need a place where we can spread out our papers and know that they will be untouched when we return. We need a place where we don't have to answer all the calls that come in, and yet we can get and receive calls when we need to.

Regardless of the kind of work we do, we need a place where we can tackle our responsibilities in peace—a place that's separate from other aspects of our life.

Reevaluate your workplace. Does it provide you with the separate space you need? If not, what do you need to do about it?

THE CHILDHOOD-ADULTHOOD PROCESS

Life begins as a quest of the child for the man and ends as a journey by the man to rediscover the child.

LAURENS VAN DER POST

Is it just that we human beings are doomed always to wish to be something that we are not, or is there another way to perceive the process of living?

What if each state of life were valued in and of itself? What if we were supported by our parenting practices to learn to be as fully in the moment as possible and to move toward adulthood as a process of unfolding, not as a goal to be accomplished?

Have you ever watched a sunrise or a sunset? These are my favorite times of day. I love the *process* of the sunrise and the sunset. There is actually no such thing as a specific sunrise or sunset (even though the papers post a "scientific time"). Sunrises and sunsets exist only as processes. The world slowly comes into daylight or comes into night. Neither shift just happens.

The same is true with growing up and growing old. If we accept the process, it is a gradual, ongoing transition; the day is always in the night, and the night always in the day. The child is always in the adult, and the adult is always in the child. From this perspective there is no such thing as a "lost childhood" or "a child within." We are all a process that at all times contains all parts of us.

Do you have the time to notice the child operating in you and the adult operating in the child? Open your perspective. Balance is participating in the whole process.

ILLUSIONS OF COMPETENCY

I'll be convinced women achieved real equality when the country is run by incompetent women.

CAPTION TO CARTOON IN *WORKING WOMAN*, AUGUST 1999

Sure we women want equality! We want an equal right to be completely incompetent and to move up the ladder as quickly as the other incompetent people around us—or do we?

Being incompetent *and* successful puts a terrible burden on us. We have to disassociate our exterior and our head from the rest of our being. We have to leave our spirituality in the closet and push ahead as if we know what we are doing and as if we are doing it well. What price is extracted (or do we extract from ourselves) when we attain this sort of equality?

When we accept incompetence in ourselves and say so, we have the opportunity to learn. When we put ourselves in the position of a learner in this life, doors open that we never knew existed, and we have the choice of walking through them or not. We never have these opportunities for learning if we are busy faking.

Faking *anything* requires us to leave ourselves and become a mask of illusionary reality. When we leave ourselves, we can never know whether it is *we* who are liked and recognized or the illusion we have created.

We are so great at so many things, why fake it anytime?

What are some of the illusions you live by? Are they worth what they cost you?

LEAVING "VICTIM"

I bid on a job that I don't have the personnel or the equipment to handle. When I got the contract, I unconsciously hired people who were not adequate for the job and ended up having to do all the work myself.

PETER

Frequently, we wake up in the middle of a mess and wonder how in the world we got there. All too often, we have put ourselves squarely in the middle, and we had absolutely no clue that we were doing it when we were doing it.

Unfortunately, most of us have learned to look outside ourselves to identify the source of the problems. We spend a lot of time and energy preparing the way to become a victim. Of course, there's no denying that others do things we don't like, things that may even be harmful to us. We have very little control over what others do and say, and we need to learn this lesson early and well. We also need to break away from popular assumptions and interpretations about our problems being " out there." When we believe we are a victim, we give our power away, resenting those who supposedly "take" it. We then become perpetrators.

Whatever the mess is, when we can sit down and carefully look at our contribution to it, we start regaining our power.

When you find yourself in the middle of a mess, sit down and examine your role in it. You'll feel better.

TURNING TO
(NOT ON) OTHERS

We must turn to each other and not on each other.

REV. JESSE JACKSON

We busy people so often do not have or take the time to deal with the feelings that build up in a normal, hectic day in a normal, hectic world.

And yet our feelings are such a precious gift. They tell us when something is not quite right. They provide us with the quick, instantaneous, surprising moments of joy in an otherwise gray day; they let us know of the love that we feel for those around us; and they let us know of danger and the need to be cautious.

Unfortunately, we have not been given the focused training, by our parents and our schools, to enable us to deal with our feelings the way we have been trained to deal with our minds.

When feelings build up inside of us, we tend to dump them on the ones nearest and dearest to us, feeling sorry later. We can do something about these behaviors and we will feel better about ourselves.

If we take a few moments of alone time before we go home from work, before others come home, or at the end of a busy day, we can learn to turn to, not on, others.

HUMILITY

Humility is being sufficient, but lacking pride in sufficiency. It is knowing grace—and knowing we did nothing to earn it. Humility is being modest, but not resigned. It is in the deepest sense—kindness.

JOYCE SEQUICHIE HIFLER

Most of us, if we think about it at all, have a great deal of confusion about humility. We confuse it with piety—especially false piety—and want nothing to do with that. Or, we see an image of self-castigating people who self-centeredly take the blame for everything, denying their own needs and accomplishments, and that doesn't look too inviting either. Yet, every spiritual path includes humility in one form or another, so we know that there must be *something* there for us.

When we look at humility as being sufficient and taking no pride in that sufficiency, we get quite a different perspective.

Being sufficient is being *enough*—not too much, not too little—just enough. Many of us have deep-seated fears of inadequacy. We fear not knowing enough to do our job well, not being good-enough parents, not being good-enough lovers, not being good-enough human beings. Yet, when we accept that we are who we are, and that as such we are enough for all the tasks presented to us, internal peace envelops us. Then, when we accept that sufficiency and peace are gifts, we know the internal balance and serenity of humility.

Take a good look at the tasks for which you have been sufficient today—and, be grateful.

EVERYDAYNESS

Zen is not some kind of excitement, but concentration on our usual everyday routine.

SHUNRYU SUZUKI

When we seek enlightenment and balance, we must look to the ordinary. It is the awareness of our presence in every little thing that we do that brings balance.

Life lived with one constant adrenaline high after another is exhausting and unreal. To approach the depth of life, one must be immersed in it. Only in our full participation in the little things can we hope to approach the infinite.

No task is too small. One is just as likely to encounter the Infinite while cleaning out the refrigerator as while sitting in a monastery meditating. Our *presence* and *participation* are what make the difference.

All too often we go for the adrenaline high to give us the illusion that we are alive and experiencing something meaningful. Whether it is at work, in sports, or in romance, the adrenaline high is the illusion. Reality is found in the everyday routine of life.

Practice being present in one activity today such as cooking, cleaning, or doing the dishes.

GIVING OURSELVES AWAY

Half the time I'm so exhausted I don't know whether I'm coming or going. It's like I'm on this nonstop merry-go-round and I can't get off. Antonio pushes himself just as hard or harder than me, and I want to keep up.

MELANIE GRIFFITH

Don't you just get exhausted reading this? I know that the term *codependence* is out of style, and yet the concept certainly is not.

One of the ways we throw ourselves completely out of balance is when we lose our own sense of what we need, get our identity through another person, and focus our energy on her or him. When we do this, we are so out of touch with ourselves that we find ourselves slowly slipping away. And when we are lost, we cannot come to others from a balanced self. Our focus is external to ourselves and we are losing ourselves in the process.

Some people believe that this focusing on the other to the exclusion of the self is love. Understandably, we hear so much about the self-sacrificing element in love. The reality, however, is that for love to exist, we have to have a self to bring to it. Those who give themselves away for the sake of love lose what they are trying to hold on to: they become a boring, uninteresting nonentity.

Giving ourselves away is never a solution.

Take a look at what you do in relationships. Do you lose yourself and give yourself away?

LAUGHING AT ONESELF

If you are willing to make yourself the butt of a joke, you become one of the guys, a human being, and people are more willing to listen to what you have to say.

LARRY WILDE

When we lose our ability to laugh at ourselves, it's a surefire indicator that we have lost our sense of balance. We have begun to take ourselves too seriously (and perhaps have even come to believe that life itself is serious). This seriousness is indicative of a severely skewed or complete loss of perspective and is therefore cause for great alarm. When we find ourselves in that dire situation, the only possible prescription (although it won't be a complete cure, because this malady is chronic and recurring in most people!) is to look at ourselves very carefully and *laugh*.

This prescription can also be used effectively when we are taking *others* too seriously, when we find them getting on our nerves. What do we need to do? We need to see how funny we are, trying to control them and buying our own delusion that each little irritating act is earth shaking.

Aren't we a hoot?!

When things start getting you down, open up to seeing what ridiculous things you are doing in the situation.

FREEDOM

*Freedom makes a huge requirement of every human being.
With freedom comes responsibility. For the person who is unwilling
to grow up, the person who does not want to carry his own weight,
this is a frightening prospect.*

ELEANOR ROOSEVELT

Living in balance contributes to our freedom. Freedom contributes to our living in balance. One without the other is not
possible.

We will never understand freedom as long as we see it as a
referent *to* or *from* something. Freedom is a state of mind and a
state of being. It occurs when we know that we are a unique creation, that we have our own connection with the life-force, and
that we have full and complete responsibility for what we do
with that gift.

The gift of freedom is the gift to make mistakes, learn from
them, and get up and try again. Freedom does not require that
we be right or even know what we are doing all the time. It simply requires that we participate in our lives and take responsibility for that participation. From this comes balance.

*Where are you with your sense of freedom and responsibili-
ty? The answers can only be found inside.*

BEING FOOLED

It is wise to remember that you are one of those who can be fooled some of the time.

LAURENCE J. PETER

Most of us like to think of ourselves as pretty savvy. We like to think that we are not easily fooled, that we have seen it all and are beyond being conned.

In some ways, though, it's a relief to know that regardless of how good we are, we are going to be fooled some of the time. That's just the way it is. Trying to delude ourselves into believing that we have moved beyond this is sheer folly of the sort that will throw us completely off balance.

When we admit that we can be fooled and acknowledge and accept it when we are, we will discover deceptions much sooner and get back to getting our life back in balance a lot more quickly.

There are some pretty good cons out there. And isn't it better to be fooled once in a while than to live with closed hearts and closed minds? When we accept who we are, we stand a better chance of accepting others as they are.

Keep open to the reality that you can be fooled, and you're less likely to be.

CRYING

Tears are a river that take you somewhere . . . Tears lift your boat off the rocks, off dry ground, carrying it down-river to someplace new, someplace better.

CLARISSA PINKOLA ESTÉS

There's nothing like a good cry to balance our lives.

Some of us are so afraid of our tears that we hold them at bay at all costs. It is still more culturally acceptable for women to cry than men (although lots of men are learning that it's okay after all), and yet, both men and women still seem to have trouble having a good cry.

I have found that some women are willing to indulge in a cry while driving along the freeway, and yet I don't really recommend it.

Every busy person knows those times when it just seems like they will either fly off the earth from centrifugal force or scream their lungs out in desperation (screaming is good, too). It is just so good to stretch out somewhere quiet and have a big old cry. Crying is *good* for us. Tears are healing. Even scientists have validated what ordinary people have known for centuries: that the body's capacity for a good cry is a great gift.

When in doubt—cry.

How long has it been since you had a good cry? Be open to the possibility.

HEALTH

Living in balance is having our bodies and teeth looked after.
ANONYMOUS

It's true, isn't it? How can we possibly live in balance if we don't take good care of our bodies and teeth?

For busy people, this may be a challenge. When we get *really* busy, we expect our bodies and teeth to take care of themselves. (We often do this with our cars and houses too.) We expect to do minimal maintenance and have all of our body parts operating at top capacity for months and months, years and years.

When our bodies start to give us warning signs that they might be in trouble, when they hint that we may be looking at a major overhaul or at lifestyle changes in the future, we get angry with them. We see the signals as an annoying personal attack. How could they *do* this to us! And just when we have an important report due (or are remodeling the house, or whatever).

Our bodies and teeth need care and understanding. They will work with us when we work with them.

How is your maintenance program for your body and teeth?
Do you need to schedule (and keep!) some appointments?

FEAR

*I have not ceased being fearful, but I have ceased to let fear control
me. I have accepted fear as a part of life—specifically the fear of
change, the fear of the unknown; and I have gone ahead despite the
pounding in my heart that says: Turn back, turn back, you'll die if
you venture too far.*

ERICA JONG

When we live our lives in fear, we are always out of balance. When we deny our fear, we are also out of balance. And, when we admit our fear and refuse to let it control us, we have the possibility of moving into balance.

Fear is normal. It is part of the human experience, a necessary survival tool. Fear provides that alertness that lets us know when our survival is threatened. Fortunately, we are rarely in situations where our life is literally threatened. That doesn't mean we've laid fear to rest. We have developed our fears to deal with more subtle situations, most of which threaten our illusion of control, our self-esteem, and our need for stasis. When we recognize this, we can relax a little and be less willing to hand our lives over to fear.

Most fear stems from lack of faith.

*Catalogue your fears. See what's underneath each of them.
This can help you get a handle on them.*

SPIRIT LAKE

This [keeping the balance between constructing our outer physical reality and creating our inner reality or selves] is why the place of the Spirit Lake, the home of the Inner Being, becomes empty and dead for so many people. They come to truly believe that the outer world is the only one worth their attention. Sooner or later they will realize their mistake.

OLGA KHARITIDI

Kharitidi writes of our task here being to create our physical reality and our inner reality, stressing that the balance between these two is important. (I would add a third element for balance—a spiritual connection with a power greater than ourselves—but that is not the issue here.)

I love the image of the Spirit Lake as the place of the Inner Being. I see my Spirit Lake as a deep pool of pure water and spirituality that I can dive into, cleansing and healing myself while infusing myself with the spiritual energy and knowledge that I need to keep balanced as I live in and cope with my physical reality.

My Spirit Lake is mine and mine alone, and I can go to it anytime, no matter where I am or what I am doing. I can be in the middle of a large, polluted city and plunge into my Spirit Lake, resurfacing with a feeling of balance.

Knowing that we can have a Spirit Lake can be a great relief.

Find your Spirit Lake. See if you have put too much emphasis on the outer world. Let your Spirit Lake give you balance.

AUTUMN

I love the fall!

ANONYMOUS

What glorious things are the seasons. There are people who scoff at living in warm places because they would never want to miss out on the change of seasons.

There is something indescribable about the sensation we feel in our bodies when we have just moved through a hot summer and one day, almost imperceptibly, we sense a change. The day or the night is just a little different. We can't even say specifically what's changed, and yet we know that fall is in the air.

That hint of fall gives us a sense of excitement, a feeling of relief. We know that we're able to trust something, that there are constants in our life: a new day will begin, and the seasons will roll on.

Then the leaves begin to turn. The chlorophyll drains out of each in turn, and we are blessed with a riot of colors that would put any fireworks display to shame. The earth explodes and skyrockets in its beauty, and we get to see and experience it. Harvest colors, foods, and celebrations invite Thanksgiving.

Get out in the fall. Experience the season. Let it flow into you.

COMPLETING OUR LISTS

One of the myths I live by is that somehow, someday, I'll get everything done.

SALLY

What a strange tendency we human beings have developed: we rush around trying to *get everything done!* We stress ourselves and others trying to complete our to-do list, knowing full well that we will always add new items to it. We live on a steady diet of the illusion that when we get everything done, *then*—and only then—will we be able to relax and do some of the things we have always wanted to do, both for ourselves and with those we love. We even perpetuate the myth that we will feel so much better after we have done everything that we will be able to relax more completely, to really have fun with family and friends. What's the matter with these people, anyway? Can't they see that we are doing all this for them?

Somehow we have failed to grasp a very basic fact: there is never a time when everything is done. That's the way life is. The relief in knowing and accepting this basic truth is immeasurable.

When we stand back and review our must-do tasks, we discover that most of them are to-do tasks that can wait.

Don't waste time trying to clear your list. Do what is important to living each step along the way.

SINGING AND DANCING

If you can walk you can dance. If you can talk you can sing.
ZIMBABWEAN PROVERB

Did you like to dance and sing when you were a kid? I did. And I still do. I wonder where the line is drawn as we are growing up—that line separating the joy of dancing and singing from the attitude that dancing and singing are not "cool." Perhaps there is no line. Perhaps we have concocted it in our imagination.

There is something about the feel of our bodies moving rhythmically through space that has a healing effect on our psyche—an effect that nothing else quite accomplishes. We begin to lose the isolation of the self and to meld our boundaries with and beyond ourselves. Nerves that have long lain dormant begin to stretch and shudder alive as our bodies reclaim themselves.

Singing is the same for us. How long has it been since you put on a favorite CD or tape and belted out old favorites with the recording artist? My observation is that even tone-deaf people love to sing. Singing stirs the soul as nothing else can. Of course, we can always *watch* and *listen* to marvelous dance and vocal concerts. And, singing and dancing don't *have* to be spectator sports.

Is there some dancing or singing activity you have always wanted to do? Try it.

WORK

The Irish hate work, not knowing what it means. I do. Work exists. It is inevitable and stark, a dull, fierce necessity.

BRENDAN KENNELLY

The Irish still hate work, it seems to me. (They're very smart that way!) At least, that has been *my* experience in Ireland. The Irish would rather be on their own time, either with family or just off doing what they like to do. There's something to be said for this attitude. Although Ireland has become the wealthiest country in the European Union, its citizens have not completely bought the European work ethic. Money is great, and yet life is more than work—that's the prevailing attitude in Ireland.

"How does this apply to me?" you ask.

Well, here's how. Often we arrange our lives around work, making it the center of our existence. We put the precious aspects of our lives—relationships, children, family, spiritual growth, personal awareness, and quiet time—on the periphery and place work solidly in the center, thus losing the perspective needed to see what is important.

When our lives are balanced, nothing is "a dull, fierce necessity."

What is you attitude toward work? Explore it honestly.

SERIOUSNESS

The world punishes us for taking it too seriously as well as for not taking it seriously enough.

AUSTIN MAC CURTAIN

As long as we are going to be punished anyway, we might as well have fun along the way.

One of the things I love about my son is that he always has fun with life. He can get bashed down by a heavy wave when he is surfing and make a comedy routine out of hightailing it for the beach and heading home. Machoism always takes a back seat to humor with him. My husband just had a disastrous trip to town, where he sat in long lines of traffic and didn't get one thing he wanted. Should he take it seriously or just have a good laugh? How important is it, anyway, in the total scheme of things?

When you get down to it, how seriously can we take what Austin Mac Curtain says? *He* seems to take it seriously. Maybe one person doing that is enough. Maybe *we* don't need to. In the larger scope of things, maybe he's willing to take the world's punishment for all of us, so we can just go bopping along. There are so many possibilities.

Don't be overly serious about the world and its possibilities for punishment. Nip that tendency in the bud.

OUR HEADS

When I finished the Ayruvedic warm-oil treatment and massage of the head, I felt as though I had eyes, ears, nose, and mouth and nothing in between. It was like all the stress I naturally have in my head had vanished, and I had an experience of free nothingness.

CONNIE

How much our heads do for us and how often we take them for granted!

I'm not talking about our thinking processes or our minds. I'm talking about our heads.

We seem to have more awareness about tension in our necks, backs, shoulders, bodies, and even feet, yet we often ignore our heads.

There are so many tiny little muscles laced across the skull—muscles that take the brunt of today's fast-paced living—and they get very little thanks for the job they do.

Connie made the above comment just after she and I had received Ayruvedic warm-oil head treatments and massages. We had been given them as gifts. She was more articulate than I was afterward. I can only say that it was one of the best gifts I have ever received. I experienced a level of relaxation and serenity that I have rarely achieved.

The simple truth is that the musculature of our skulls is on duty a lot and therefore needs considerable attention. Noticing, respecting, and caring for our heads is a great balancer in life.

Find a place to get either a head massage or an oil treatment with massage for your hair. If that's not possible, trade head massages with a friend or spouse. You won't regret it.

TRUTH

Truth has no special time of its own. Its hour is now—always.
ALBERT SCHWEITZER

Some of us live our lives in search of truth, believing that someday we will happen upon it and it will illuminate us forever. The strange thing about truth is that it is not one big thing. Truth is a conglomeration of little things that may go unnoticed at the time. Truth expands and constricts depending upon our ability to perceive it.

Often, we try to make truth too small, and in doing so we eliminate it. We suspect that our children are using drugs and announce that we are going to get to the "real truth." In the process, we may forget the larger truth—that we love them mightily and they love us.

We spend some time with a hospitalized neighbor who is getting a bit forgetful. When she says that her husband bought her the new robe that we just bought her, we watch as the nurse tries to get her to see the "truth"—that her husband has been dead for many years. A gift is a gift. Does it really matter?

We search for truth about *things* so diligently that we often pass up the daily opportunity to experience the truth about *living.*

The big truths are also little. It's a beautiful day (no matter what the weather is). Today we have what we need (even if it is not all we want!). Today we are learning about living in all we do.

What is the truth of your "now"? Seeing it can return you to balance.

LEGACIES

Memory is the diary we all carry about with us.
MARY H. WALDRIP

Perhaps the most important thing we can do in this life is to do no harm. Down deep, we all probably want to be (and be seen as) loving, caring, and concerned people. We don't want to leave the legacy of having been an unkind person.

As we try to build and support this image of ourselves, we often overlook the role of memory. Every person we touch unconsciously carries a "diary" within. Our behaviors are the scribes in that diary. All too often the memories are written in permanent ink regardless of our wishes or those of the person in whose diary our behaviors are being written.

It is up to us to determine what is written in that diary. We are responsible for our own behaviors. When we choose to act out, be dishonest, con the unwary, or be destructive, the diaries of those we care about most are recording those acts, and it is difficult to tear out the pages or erase the inscriptions. It behooves us to be conscious of our words and our behaviors and to pause before we act on unloving or destructive thoughts.

When we practice doing no harm, we contribute to a legacy we are proud to claim.

Be more aware this week of what you say and do. See if your are shaping the legacy you want to contribute.

RIGHT ACTION

Do right always. It will give you satisfaction in life.

WOVOKA

Right action can be an elusive concept. What may seem right in the spur of the moment may, after a few minutes of reflection, be revealed as completely the wrong thing to do. (It's good to reflect on decisions, if possible.) And what may have seemed wrong or at least unpopular in the moment may turn out to be the best decision you have ever made.

Doing right, in the best spirit of the phrase, means using a combination of our intellect, intuition, and experience to make decisions that are right for both ourselves and others. If we are clear and in touch with our spirituality, we will feel good about decisions that are good for others as well as ourselves. Whenever we decide something that benefits only ourselves or those near and dear to us, satisfaction fades rapidly (in spite of how "smart" that decision may have seemed at the time).

Somewhere, someplace, there is a celestial measuring rod for right action, and its reflection resides in us.

Get a little blank book that you can carry with you at all times. Take time every day to write down some of the things you did right that day, remembering that some of the most "right" things may have looked "wrong" to you or others at the time.

UNDERSTANDING
WITH YOUR HEART

Remember, Elizabeth Anne, we never really know what is going on inside another person to make them act the way they do. Try to understand that they have their reasons.

MANILLA LONGAN

My mother was a natural healer of people. She always tried to teach me that we can never completely understand another person, though we can accept that they have their reasons. She didn't interpret. She didn't analyze or figure out. She "understood" with her heart.

Over the years, I have come to see how destructive it is to interpret another person. The arrogance, judgmentalism, and harshness of interpretation go a long way toward destroying relationships. Even when our interpretations make sense and are based on "facts," they may have absolutely nothing to do with genuine reality.

When we analyze or try to figure out other people, we have made them an object to be observed. We have left behind our oneness, our connectedness with them; we have elevated ourselves above them and become uncaring. We are trying to do their work for them.

When we understand with our heart, we see that others have "reasons" we aren't privy to that lie behind their behaviors. We can care for them as people like ourselves—people who are struggling to learn from life.

Set up a red-flag system to alert you whenever you begin to analyze or interpret others. Stop yourself and instead try to understand with your heart.

DEEPER LEARNING

The person who knows "how" will always have a job. The person who knows "why" will always be his boss.

DIANE RAVITCH

We are a lot smarter than some people think we are.

We live in a technological age where the demand for technicians is great and companies are willing to pay excellent salaries (with benefits!) for good technicians. Fortunately, however, good salaries and benefits just aren't enough. We want more out of life. We want to know something. We want to explore the whys of what we do—even the whys of life. We want to experience the creativity of learning, learning, learning. We want to move and stretch and expand our minds and knowledge. There is so much to explore. Why not explore it?

Just as soon as we get the "how" down, we are ready to go deeper. It's great to learn how to do something, whether how to make it through an exotic recipe or how to carve a beautiful wooden door. And, as soon as we become expert at the recipe, we want to try variations and explore why certain herbs and spices produce a better result than others. And as soon as we finish the door, we may take up carving as a hobby. We want to know even more about woods and tools and possibilities.

Human beings are like this. We get off balance when we stop on the tip of the iceberg, and we thrive when we have vast knowledge about something that intrigues us.

Give in to that urge to know more. Find books, people, and situations that can help you. It's enlivening.

IMAGINATIONS

Without imagination, there is no goodness, no wisdom.
MARIE VON EBNER-ESCHENBACH

What wonderful things our imaginations are. When we were children, imagination was so easy. We had imaginary playmates, we saw sailing ships in the clouds, and we pretended in our play, making up characters, plots, and roles. What happened?

As adults, often the only time our imaginations come into play is when we make up stories about how someone is feeling toward us or thinks about us. "I'm sure she hates me; she just seemed strange when I ran into her the other day." "He's just out to get me." Perhaps our imagination is just so out of practice that it has taken a negative turn.

We can fix that. Imagination just asks us to look at the whole range of options. It can be very ordinary. For example, we have a lovely old pine corner cabinet that we bought for our house. It looks as if it had been made (one hundred years ago!) expressly for our corner. After doing some remodeling, we decided to get window quilts to conserve energy, but unfortunately the top of the cabinet and the roller for the window quilt needed the same space on the wall. What to do? Cut off part of the cabinet? Absolutely not. Opt not to install the window quilt? Absolutely not. Shift the cabinet out of the corner? No. Put it in another corner? Not possible. It was time for imagination. Raise up the cabinet and build a storage shelf with a door underneath it so both could fit. Of course!

Get reacquainted with your creative imagination. Try using it to solve simple problems around the house.

THE NEWS MEDIA

I get jangled and depressed when I read newspapers and watch the news.

LOUISE

The media have changed over the last fifty years. The focus has shifted from dispensing information to accessing worry and adrenaline. Rare is the story of someone quietly living his or her life in a serene and happy way—unless, of course, there is an "angle" attached. Rare is the passing on of helpful information—unless there is a hidden agenda of manipulating our perceptions. More and more space and time is devoted to business and technology, and less and less to "human interest." We almost never see anything about the singular heroic people who are quietly working to save the wetlands, facilitate knowledge about reconciliation with the wolves, or plant seeds of healing.

How can we live in balance when the sources we turn to for information are so unbalanced?

Give up newspapers and the other media for a week. Spend the time you would usually have devoted to these endeavors either with family and friends or reading something meditative. See what happens. Find other ways of getting information.

BEING OF SERVICE

Serving God is doing good to man. But praying is thought an easier service and is therefore more generally chosen.

BENJAMIN FRANKLIN

So many of us would like to be of service, if we just knew how. And we're daunted by the prospect. Actual service is so *personal*. It's so *hands on*. And, let's admit it, some of us feel shy and inadequate when it comes to doing service directly. We'd rather give money—a good thing and not very personal. We'd rather pray—more sanitized and again not personal. We feel better after both. Still, nothing can substitute for doing something for someone else—personally.

There is something about this particular activity that adjusts the vertebrae of our very being. We don't have to do anything big. We can build our service muscles through small tasks, such as helping an elderly person, picking up trash, letting someone who is in a hurry go before us in the checkout line. Regardless of what we do, service is a prayer, and we need all the prayers we can get to balance our lives.

Do some kind of service every day, and you will start seeing opportunities for more. Service is kindness in action.

STANDING OUT

Life has taught me that it is not for our faults that we are disliked and even hated but for our qualities.

BERNARD BERENSON

How dangerous it is to be excellent! We live in a world where mediocrity means safety. Women, especially, have learned that it is very dangerous to stick our heads above the crowd. There are always others who would like to take a swing at any target, heads included. Sadly, we have often learned the hard way that the strongest swingers of the beheading sword are other women, although some men likewise jump at the chance.

Somewhere, somehow, we have learned that the safest position we can take is in back, down low. We sit on our power and try not to let others (even ourselves!) see it. We may have the *illusion* of safety and the *feeling* of being a clogged-up sewer pipe.

Claiming our power may be dangerous, and . . . it sure is fun!

Sit down and write out ways you have stifled your power. See which ones you are ready to change, and start with one today.

WORRY AND CONTROL

Worry never robs tomorrow of its sorrow; it only saps today of its strength.

A.J. CRONIN

How often do we rob ourselves of the balance in our lives by indulging in worry? Worry is so easy to justify that it has become one of our favorite national pastimes. Some people even believe that they *owe* it to their friends and family to worry about them.

Worry is one of the main ways we unbalance ourselves. The other day I was standing in line at the airport to get a ticket changed. The line was moving *very* slowly, and yet it was clear that the people at the desk were doing the best they could. As we waited, the men in front of me worked themselves into hissy fits. Never have I heard such a cacophony of sighs and mumbles (quickly escalating to loud remarks). The men repeatedly marched up to the counter to tell the agent how urgent *their* plight was, even after the agent had told them that they could not possibly catch the flight they wanted. They firmly believed that the agent could solve the problem that they were creating within themselves. It was so clear that they were working themselves up and only *they* could return themselves to balance. Only when they let themselves realize that they cannot control people, places, or things—only when they let go of their illusion of control—will they feel relaxed, serene, and balanced.

When you find yourself starting to worry about something, stop, check out what you are trying to control, let go, relax, and return to balance.

PREPAREDNESS

God sneezed. What could I say to Him?

HENNY YOUNGMAN

Aren't there just those times when we are at a loss for words? Our life experiences have just not prepared us for this or that particular occasion. Well, yes, these are unbalancing times. My heavens, how we love to be prepared. Somewhere along the line we have picked up the not-so-subtle message that the way to safety is preparedness. The Boy Scouts are prepared. The Girl Scouts are prepared. Grand universities and colleges survive on the myth of preparedness. Yet there are always those occasions for which we are not prepared.

Maybe the ultimate preparedness is the ability to hang loose in every situation. Maybe the issue is to have such an intimate, strong relationship with God that when God sneezes, we can simply say, "Need a tissue?"

Preparedness won't save us. Presence might.

Check to see if your illusions about the need for prepared-ness are limiting your life. How can you use your skills and let go at the same time?

KINDNESS

A little kindness from person to person is better than a vast love for all humankind.

RICHARD DEHMEL

Sometimes it seems as if our world is becoming more and more abstract and in the process less and less intimate. City living and impersonal, isolated suburban homes make it easy to have an abstract concept of being a loving person without having to test that hypothesis outside a very close circle of family and friends.

Kindness is the heart stretching itself and opening up clogged arteries before they know they have a problem. Kindness is the simple, unnoticed act of being present to the context of our daily lives. Kindness is the letting go of fixed societal procedures to reach across the chasm of isolation and touch another being. Kindness is a stretching, a movement, a touching that is more felt than thought.

Our practice of kindness shows us a self that we can come to like and even love. We are all capable of kindness.

Practice kindness with a stranger.

CHILDREN

The reason most people have kids is because they get pregnant.
BARBARA KINGSOLVER

There are so many reasons for having children—most of which are probably unknown even to us. Some say that we are slaves to our hormones and the procreation of our species. Others have children to carry on the family name or genes. Still others have children as the last great unexplored frontier, when they have done everything else. For themselves. To love and be loved. For the experience. To save or justify a marriage. Because they love children. Some because they want to take the responsibility to support and nurture another life. Here's another perspective: perhaps we are given children to throw our lives out of balance. Children certainly do that. From the moment they are conceived, they send our illusion of order and control flying. Our need for immaculate clothing and studied chic quickly goes out the window as well, with the arrival of spit-up and yellow-green poo. Our ability to organize and feed our belief that we are in charge goes up in smoke as chaos takes over. Our illusion that we can predict and know the future evaporates with sore throats and the fussiness of teething.

Children bring us the gift of unbalancing our lives so that we can let go of our belief in making our world static. God bless them!

Perhaps now would be a good time to change perspective and see disruptions and unplanned events as positives that can help us grow.

OVEREXTENDING

When I start brushing my teeth while I shower, it's a clue that I'm overextended.

CONNIE

Aren't we funny? We believe that we are "saving time" when we crowd necessary activities in on top of each other. We nurse the illusion that "efficiency" is being able to do several tasks at the same time while attending to none of them. We rob ourselves of the awareness of what we are doing while trying to find ways to do more.

Ironically, in our attempt to overlap activities and accomplish as much as we can in as little time as possible, we increase the stress we feel, which results in our being less efficient and making more mistakes.

But . . . do we stop to look at the results of our rushing and overlapping? No! We plunge on, trusting our preconceived notions about what is efficient and what is not.

Now you have to admit . . . that's funny!

What are your red flags that let you know you are overextending yourself? Write them down and share them with someone else so that the truth is out.

INTERDEPENDENCE

Things derive their being and nature by mutual dependence and are nothing in themselves.

NAGARJUNA

Are you ready to part with your illusion that you exist by yourself and stand alone in the universe? So many self-made women and men fall prey to the illusion that everything they do they do themselves and that the path to their success was made only by them.

This is a costly illusion. In order to maintain it, we have to forget the women who gave birth to us, the ones who raised us—the people who taught us—by their example and by the opposite of their example. We have to forget the pains caused by those who have loved us and by those who have refused to love us. We have to bury the memories of the animals, rocks, and trees that shared their essence with us when we needed it most. We cannot let ourselves know those unknown forces that have participated at levels beyond comprehension. We have to ignore those who make our clothes, build our houses, grow our food, and prepare it so that we can move toward self-actualization.

Only in knowing our dependence, independence, counter-dependence, and interdependence can we balance ourselves.

Go over the list above, add some categories of your own, and acknowledge those who have contributed to your something-ness.

ENTHUSIASM

You will do foolish things but do them with enthusiasm.

COLETTE

Ah, enthusiasm! It is not just something reserved for children, the unsophisticated, and the insane. Enthusiasm is a normal human response to the joy, excitement, and surprises of life. Why not feel it?

Enthusiasm is a balancer. It sparks life and then renews it when it fades. Enthusiasm gets the juices flowing. It turns the ordinary into the extraordinary and opens the door for more and more extraordinaries.

Enthusiasm is infectious. We can be hanging around like a bunch of old couch potatoes, and one enthusiastic person can get us moving. It's good to get the juices flowing.

Where in the world did we get the impression that enthusiasm is "uncool"? Where did we get the idea that we are too old for it? Where did we get the notion that enthusiastic people are trying to manipulate us or are unreal? Forget it! Get over it!

Each of us still has large wells of enthusiasm within us, though they may be buried deep and hidden well.

Dig a little.

Nurture those things that feed your enthusiasm.

LOVING DREAMS

I will not be involved with the dreams of angry men.
HMONG VILLAGER

How profound! How much of our dis-ease and lack of balance comes from being "involved with the dreams of angry men" (or women!), whether those dreamers are ourselves, our families, our co-workers, our bosses, or our politicians.

We have a choice about participating in the dreams of angry people: all by ourselves we can begin to build the dreams of a *loving* people. Down deep, most of us want to be loving people. We want to experience ourselves as loving, and we want to share that love with others.

Some of us may be afraid of the risk. In days past, we may have been hurt, rejected, ignored, or even punished for loving. That's okay. We can handle it. Surely we learned something from it. Even if we have had these experiences and feel that we need to protect ourselves somewhere deep within, we have the ability to dream the dreams of a loving person and to participate in the dreams of other loving people.

What are your dreams as a loving person? Are you in touch with them, or do you need to do a bit of seeking? Feel free to seek.

GIFTS

When one's heart is glad, he gives away gifts. It [the potlatch] was given to us by our Creator to be our way of doing things, we who are Indians. The potlatch was given to us to be our way of expressing joy.

AGNES ALFRED

What a pleasure it is to give gifts—something *from* the heart, something *to* the heart.

Most of us take flowers or a bottle of wine when we are invited to dinner. Yet how frequently do we let ourselves participate in *spontaneous* gift-giving? How often do we keep our eyes and our ears open to others so that we know them well enough to pick out just the right little present, one that will let their heart soar? It's great fun to see surprise and pleasure bursting forth on the face of someone we like and love. How much more fun it is to give something spontaneously to someone we've just met. Our hearts have to be very large to give gifts, and they grow with each gift given.

We don't have to "give until it hurts." We don't have to worry ourselves about what to give. We can just let the spontaneity be our guide.

Gifts are fun to receive and fun to give. Gift-giving restores balance.

Cultivate your spontaneous gift-giving.

QUIET TIME

I need quiet time every day. It's just like vitamin C: my body and my being can't store it up. I need regular doses.

WAYNE

So often, those of us who do too much collapse into a week-end retreat or a sick day. We sleep all day or all weekend and believe that we have had our quiet time for a while.

We need quiet time *every* day, and it is up to us to arrange it. Let me put this in big, bold letters: NO ONE ELSE WILL SEE THAT WE HAVE QUIET TIME. WE HAVE TO DO IT OURSELVES.

Our beings need a daily dose of quiet time to gather ourselves.

Some people choose to get up an hour or a half-hour earlier than they usually do. This is a good approach, because it's wise to take the time for oneself first and then enter into the process of getting ready for the day. Otherwise, we might lose the opening. Most people find that quiet time energizes them so much that they don't miss the sleep.

Others lock themselves in the bathroom for a few minutes at home or at work—it usually pays off. Still others take quiet time mini-breaks—moments of reflection while sitting at the computer, while washing dishes, while taking a walk.

Quiet time is like food, water, and air. We need it for survival.

Are you designing moments of quiet time in your life? Do you have enough? What do you need to do?

CHEERFULNESS

Cheerfulness keeps up a kind of daylight in the mind, and fills it with a steady and perpetual serenity.

JOSEPH ADDISON

As Beverly Sills says, "I can't be happy every day, but I can be cheerful."

Being cheerful is a choice that leads to happiness. Gloom and doom have a hard time surviving around a cheerful person. Besides, being cheerful is fun.

A cheerful person accepts life on life's terms and finds the good in those terms. No matter what, if we try hard enough we can find some good in almost everything and everyone. Looking for good is what cheerfulness does.

When we realize that nothing is more important than our own sense of inner peace and the happiness of our loved ones and ourselves, cheerfulness comes naturally. When we achieve that sense of inner peace, our needs, desires, and concerns diminish; those that remain fall into their appropriate places.

Cheerfulness is possible when we accept reality and know that whatever the present is, the future will be different.

Perspective invites cheerfulness.

Practice cheerfulness in all your affairs.

MINDING OUR OWN BUSINESS

Some of 'em so expert on mindin' folks' business dat dey kin look at de smoke comin' out yo' chimbley and tell yuh what yuh cookin'!
ZORA NEALE HURSTON

Let's take a look at nosiness. Now of course, no people who do too much *really* have the time to be nosy. Still, this may be a problem for some of us. If so, it can be one of the things that gets us off balance. Let's take a look at it.

There is an unlimited number of people who are more than willing to involve us in their business. We get many invitations to try to solve issues that have absolutely nothing to do with us. The invitations are always beautiful hooks that flatter us and imply that we have great knowledge, experience, strength, or beauty. And remember, just because someone shows us a hook, we don't have to fling ourselves onto it.

We need to get a new vision of what is our business and then we need to learn to mind our own business. Being overly involved in situations others have set up for themselves, for their *own* learning, can be a quagmire. We need to resist the temptation to jump in and help, especially when no one has even asked for our help.

When we redefine what is our business, we may discover that the scope is much smaller than we had imagined.

Practice minding your own business.

STRESS

Stress is an ignorant state. It believes that everything is an emergency.

NATALIE GOLDBERG

Some say that stress is inherent in modern life—probably true. What they don't say is that we inflict some of the stress upon ourselves and that we have a good deal of influence over the amount and the intensity of that self-inflicted stress.

For example, one of our greatest causes of stress is drama. Something happens, and we blow it all out of proportion, making it out to be the end of the world. I recently was a houseguest of a woman who took that approach the entire time I was there. Try as I might, I found it very difficult to stay centered and protect myself from her constant barrage of energy. I felt exhausted when I left. I didn't get into the drama, and yet I found it tiring to be around.

Another area where we stress ourselves unduly is driving. Almost imperceptibly we find ourselves competing when we drive. Is it really worth it? We can learn to be less aggressive when we drive.

We also stress ourselves by trying to accomplish things that just aren't ready to be done. We fail to recognize that *our* schedule doesn't match that of everyone and everything else. All too often things unfold as they will, oblivious to our intentions. When we recognize this, our lives become easier.

Much of our stress is of our own creation.

Look at the ways you create stress for yourself. See what you can change in the ways you approach these situations. Be alert to the signals that stress is building.

MOODS

I never thought of myself as a moody person and I do have moods.
LOUISE

Most of us don't think of ourselves as being moody, and yet almost all of us, unless we are completely out of touch with ourselves, do have moods.

It's not that moods are wrong. They just *are.* They are as much a part of us as anything else. We certainly don't have to get rid of them, though we *do* need to learn how to live with them well and maybe even how to recognize what they are meant to teach us.

As we learn to recognize our moods, we can get friendly with them. They're just moods, after all. Sometimes, for seemingly no good reason, we just start feeling grinchy and a little mean (not at all like us, of course *and*—there it is). We need to honor and respect these times. A bad mood may be the opening into an important awareness that is ready to come up for our learning.

Most of all, we need to refrain from dumping our moods on those we love. They'll only be hurt, and we'll feel bad about ourselves. Once we learn to see our moods and honor them (not deny them), we are able to warn others of thunderclouds on the horizon and clearly let them know that the mood has nothing to do with them. We can assure them that whatever it is, it is something bubbling up that we have the opportunity to learn from. By honoring and respecting our moods in this way, we can bring balance to our situation.

How do you handle your moods? Do you recognize them and honor them? Where you are in accepting your moods will determine how you respond to them.

SELF-EXPLORATION

There are three vertical levels in every individual: natural, spiritual, and heavenly.

EMANUEL SWEDENBORG

So many great teachers and spiritual approaches have talked about three levels in the human. Swedenborg talked of the natural, the spiritual, and the heavenly. Freud talked about the id, the ego, and the superego. The Huna tradition talks about the physical, the lower self, and the higher self. Christianity talks about the physical life, hell, and heaven. No matter what makes sense to us or what path we choose to follow, there seems to be a general consensus that we are more than just this conscious self (and thus have to deal with more than just this conscious self).

We have glimpses of these other levels. We have flashes, intuitions, dreams, random thoughts, and random awarenesses, so we realize that there is something going on at some other level. The fact that we do things that we don't understand and have feelings that we can't explain reinforces that conclusion.

What exciting possibilities! We have unknowns! Better yet, we have unknowns in ourselves! We have the unlimited possibility of self-exploration. We cannot do this exploration only with our intellect. We need our minds, spirits, feelings, intuitions, whispers, dreams, and flashes before we can even begin.

Our life is such an opportunity.

Give yourself the time and attention you need to explore your universes. It's good if you can be open to everything that is available to you.

PREPARATION

[Preparation] is the be-all of good trial work. Everything else—felicity of expression, improvisational brilliance—is a satellite around the sun. Thorough preparation is that sun.

LOUIS NIZER

Preparation is a good balancer. I'm not talking about the kind of preparation that people who do to much sometimes do—the last-minute, frantic, and obsessive kind that never feels like enough. I'm talking about steady (even plodding), reasonable, thorough preparation.

Preparing for something—anything—can be fun in itself. We can explore the options, gather data, discover surprises, and create new ideas and approaches. We can glean information where we thought there was none and move into areas of research never before envisioned. Good preparation is an adventure and a discovery.

Good preparation is also much more. When we are prepared, we feel more balanced and more secure. When we are prepared, we can allow ourselves to be more spontaneous—more improvisational, if you will. In that mode, we're more likely to be able adequately, even creatively, to deal with new and surprising information.

Preparation is a security blanket.

How do you approach preparation for most things? Could you do more to support your being calm and centered when you go into a potentially stressful situation? Do your homework.

SMILING

A smile is a light on your face to let someone know you are at home.
ANONYMOUS

We're talking about a genuine smile here, not something pasted on your face. Everyone can see through a phony smile. There's no light in it.

But ah, the light in a genuine smile! It can make the most homely face seem beautiful, the most uninteresting person fascinating.

A smile is good for everyone around it. It is an invitation to radiance, a proclamation of aliveness, and a gesture of peace. A genuine smile can open doors and hearts and spread light where darkness has prevailed.

A smile is also good for the smiler. When we smile, our head relaxes and the muscles used for thinking and stress have to let go a little. Once they loosen their grip, a whole chain reaction is started, and ease creeps in where only dis-ease had reigned.

A smile is also cheap. In fact, it doesn't cost a thing, and the results are far-reaching.

Go ahead: let yourself smile more.

COMPARISONS

A humility that begins with the acceptance of self as imperfect will not be interested in judging others: "To be humble is not to make comparisons."

ERNEST KURTZ AND KATHERINE KETCHAM

Who in the world thought up comparisons? And, why are we taught to think in comparisons? Has anything good ever come from comparing ourselves to other people and they to us? Think about it! Someone always loses. Since each one of us is perfectly unique, we are always comparing apples and oranges—so what sense does it make?

There is no way to be perfectly happy with yourself or with others if you routinely compare yourself to someone else. There is no way to be happy with your partner or lover if you compare that person to someone else. There is no way to be happy and humble if you compare your job with someone else's. And, there is no way to be happy and humble with something you have produced if you compare it with anything someone else has produced. Comparisons are deadly, and they're rarely, if ever, useful in the essence of living.

Let comparing be one of your red-flag activities. When you start doing it, stop to ask yourself if it's what you really want to do.

HOME MAINTENANCE

My life got a lot easier when I realized that there would always be something that needed to be done with the house.

CHUCK

As a young housewife and professional woman, I had the illusion that after I got my house just the way I wanted it (which, of course, would take some time and effort), it would stay that way forever. Nothing in my training and education had prepared me for the reality that loose covers wear out, walls need to be painted and repainted, and plates break and chip.

My husband approached what he perceived as his responsibility to the house the same way. He thought that he would get the initial maintenance or remodeling done, and that would be it.

With these attitudes, we both soon began to feel like victims of our house. We actually began to have anger toward our "dream house," which threw the household out of balance.

When we stopped viewing the house as a series of big projects that would be finished (at which time we could relax) and began to see it as a living, moving, changing organism that was very important to the quality of our lives, and with which we had an ongoing relationship, our lives became more relaxed. We could work with our home and maintain it just as we maintained our bodies, our relationships, and our spirituality.

Check out your perspective with respect to home maintenance. Do you need to initiate some changes to make your life better?

ANGER

It's my rule never to lose me temper till it would be detrimental to keep it.

SEAN O'CASEY

There are two important points to be emphasized here: (1) trying not to lose our temper and (2) there are times when it is detrimental to keep anger in check.

Anger is not a negative emotion. It is just an emotion. Sometimes we get angry. Sometimes our anger is justified, and sometimes it's not. But that's not the point. The real issue is what we do with our temper.

Lashing out when we are angry can be detrimental to ourselves and others. Holding our tempers in can be detrimental to ourselves and others as well.

We need to have safe places to vent our anger, releasing it in such a way that it is not directed at ourselves or anyone else. Often when we react strongly, there is some older, deeper issue that is being triggered that we have the opportunity to resolve.

I suggest having a mat in a safe place where we can stretch out and let the feelings roll. Clearing our temper is like having a good celestial enema.

Arrange a safe place in your home where you can stretch out and let feelings out.

HAVING ENOUGH

I've never been poor, only broke. Being poor is a frame of mind. Being broke is only a temporary situation.

MIKE TODD

We can have great monetary wealth and still be poor. We can have no money at all and not be poor.

I've always had difficulty with the concept of "the poor." Although I've been there myself many times, and grew up in what some would consider a "poor" family, I've never *felt* poor. Even without money, our lives were rich. I have also seen this in others who had no money.

Don't take me wrong. I like money, and when I have it, I enjoy it. And, there's a deeper issue at stake here. Seeing others as poor takes a certain arrogance. Often those who see others (or themselves) this way are in need of what those they define as poor have.

If being poor is a frame of mind, this frame of mind is one that says that we don't have enough and will probably believe that we never will have enough. From this perspective, "enough" is also a frame of mind and from this frame of mind, enough never really exists.

Having enough means that somewhere deep inside of us we have an awareness of the abundance around us. Enough stems from an awareness of a valuing of what we have and does not focus on what we *don't* have. Having enough is knowing that we ourselves are enough and can live well with what we have each moment of our lives.

Are you caught in an enough/not enough struggle in any area of your life? Tackle it by making daily gratitude lists.

THE WEATHER

Never has the earth been so lovely or the sun so bright, as today . . .
NIKINAPI

Never has the earth been so lovely as on this beautiful, rainy day. Never has the earth been so lovely as on this beautiful, snowy day. Never has the earth been so lovely as on this beautiful, foggy day. The earth is so lovely.

The American Indians in their wisdom knew that the earth needs all kinds of days in order to prosper and be healthy. If we had only sunny days, the earth would be parched. If we had only rainy days, nothing would grow. Like the earth, we need balance to grow and experience life.

We human beings also need all kinds of days to experience the fullness of our lives. Remember when you were a child and a heavy snowfall pushed the schools to declare a snow day? Wasn't it a gift from heaven? A "free" day. It was too cold or snowy to go to school, and we could play in it or snuggle down at home and just relax.

The weather and the days affect us. Sometimes rainy days invite us to pull inside and do quiet work. Sunny days can energize. If we let ourselves respond to the days given us, each is beautiful and each can call forth a response in us that is necessary for us.

We can be grateful for each day as it is and can start right now.

MARRIAGE

It takes a long time to really be married. One marries many times at many levels within a marriage. If you have more marriages than you have divorces within the marriage, you're lucky and you stick it out.

RUBY DEE

Balance in a marriage or other intimate relationship is never achieved by trying to get the relationship just the way you want it and then keeping it that way. Marriage is a process in which each spouse has the option of participating. When we try to build the relationship to some "finished" state and then keep it static there, we are inviting death into what should be a moving, changing process. The only way to keep a process that we truly care about alive is to participate in it. Balance is participation. A good marriage merges participation with forgiveness and caring. Stasis has no place here.

When we truly participate, approaching the relationship out of our spirituality, we feel love. When we move out of our spirituality, miracles are possible.

Take a look at ways you might be trying to make your marriage or other intimate relationship static. What do you need to do to move away from control and toward greater participation?

STRESS TOLERANCE

Our current level of stress will be exactly that of our tolerance of stress.

RICHARD CARLSON

I remember years ago when I was researching workaholism, making what was to me at the time a startling discovery. Workaholics were using stress-reducing activities and health-enhancing approaches to support their workaholism! Under the guise of working out to reduce stress and take care of their bodies, they were getting fitter so that they could work harder. Under the guise of changing their diets and eating better to be healthier, they were using a good diet to support their addiction. They were just increasing their tolerance. They were not dealing with the real issues.

Somewhere along the line, we have bought into the myth that increasing our tolerance of stress is a good thing—and so we deal with progressively increasing levels of stress.

What if we began to *decrease* our tolerance for stress? Would we then have less stress in our lives? I believe so. Would this then be good for our bodies, minds, and souls? I believe so.

Are you ready to decrease your level of stress tolerance and hence your level of stress? Start by spending more time in nature and having more quiet time.

MODELING CHANGE

I tried to leave work on time several days and I just couldn't do it.
ROLAND

I once knew a businesswoman who decided that she wanted to run a sane organization. One of the steps she took in that direction was to encourage her employees to work carefully and hard during the workday and then to leave the office on time, preferably not taking anything home with them. Then she made a difficult discovery: her employees wouldn't leave on time unless she left on time. And they insisted on taking work home with them as long as she took work home with her.

If she wanted her employees to change and approach work more sanely, she had to do the same thing. Her life changed dramatically.

Words are great, and most people don't believe them when the speaker's actions are different from the words. Modeling change is so different from talking about it. Don't tell me: show me!

Focus on one change you would like to make in your work or home environment and model it.

WHOLENESS

A person who believes . . . that there is a whole of which one is a part, and that in being a part one is whole: such a person has no desire whatever, at any time, to play God. Only those who have denied their being yearn to play at it.

URSULA K. LeGUIN

There is such comfort in knowing that there is a wholeness in all creation and that we are a part of that creation! Fortunately, this wholeness is not an intellectual concept. It is a *felt* concept; and when it is felt and experienced, one can never again completely leave the knowledge and comfort of being a part of a larger whole. This feeling of connectedness is not one that we can conjure up at will. Ironically, though, it is always there inside of us; we have only to stop long enough to open ourselves up to the memory of it.

We are not looking for something we don't know. We are looking for something that our DNA has known for centuries. We have only to rediscover it.

Sometimes we try to avoid the awareness of being part of a larger whole because we want to assert our uniqueness; we are afraid of losing our individuality. Not to worry: we become more ourselves as we feel our belonging to the all-that-is.

You can't make this awareness of wholeness happen, and yet you can be open to it. Many people seem to have this experience and knowing in nature, perhaps while gazing at the stars. Try to make time for these activities.

CONDEMNING OTHERS

Someone has said that it requires less mental effort to condemn than to think.

EMMA GOLDMAN

Condemning others is a subtle and destructive process. Whenever we are tempted to indulge in condemnation, we need to stop, take a deep breath, and ask ourselves if it is really worth it.

When we are involved in the process of condemning others (or engaged in its milder form: disapproval), we are usually so enmeshed in the activity that we don't take the time to stop, step back, and see the damage we are doing to ourselves.

At the very least, we are taking what could be a positive moment in our lives and plunging ourselves into negativity. We are focusing on someone outside of ourselves and generating judgmentalism. In order to indulge in this activity, we have to leave ourselves. Is it worth it?

Whenever we condemn or disapprove, we plunge into the negative, leaving ourselves in the process. It may take a long time to crawl out again.

Whenever you start to enter into the condemning/disapproval process, stop to ask yourself if this is what you really want to do. You'll be glad you did.

PRAYER AND DRAMA

Any concern too small to be turned into a prayer is too small to be made into a burden.

CORRIE TEN BOOM

Here is a good measuring stick for balancing our lives: if our worries are too small for prayer, they don't deserve to be worried over. If they are big enough for prayer, we can utter a brief few words, turn them over, and let them go. Either way, there is no need to carry a burden.

So many of the issues in our lives need not be issues. This does not mean that we don't have issues. Of course we do: that's what life is—having issues, facing them, and learning from them. The *issues* are not the issue. *We* are the issue.

We have many choices about the way we respond to any given incident, but the incident is the same no matter how we respond. It just is. When we respond with drama, adrenaline, overkill, and excessive energy, our response is guaranteed to exacerbate the situation. When we choose this response and then wonder why we have a mess, we feel like victims. When we feel like victims, we want to get revenge on the person who *made* us feel this way. And so on . . .

If we just take a deep breath at the beginning and ask ourselves if we want to make it a game or drama (or enter the drama if it has already started), develop it into a burden, or sigh and utter a short prayer of willingness to react another way or not at all, our lives get smoother.

Try it!

PAIN

I imagine one of the reasons people cling to their hates so stubbornly is because they sense, once hate is gone, they will be forced to deal with pain.

JAMES BALDWIN

Trying to cover up our pain throws us out of balance. When we feel deep pain, we often substitute emotions that put the focus outside ourselves and distract us from facing those feelings that would bring balance back to our lives.

Fear, hatred, anger, and resentment are means by which we try to distract ourselves from dealing with the empty pits we sometimes sense deep in ourselves—pits that seem terribly frightening.

Yet, how can we know who we truly are, and become all that we can be, unless we are willing to plunge beneath the obvious and confront our pain?

If we allow ourselves to move beneath the surface, our inner beings won't let us be overwhelmed by what's there. When we take time to experience and work through our pain on a feeling-level, our lives become lighter.

Take some time alone and tell your inner being that you are ready to deal with old pains. (Don't lie to it!) Prepare yourself for a great adventure.

INTUITION

Don't listen to friends when the Friend inside you says "Do this!"
MAHATMA GANDHI

What a difficult time we have trusting our hunches and intuition! Our training that our intuitive mind is not "logical" or "rational" goes very deep.

Some of us have become so divorced from our intuition, having been told that it is not "scientific," that we have tried to shut off that quiet voice of knowing within ourselves—a voice that is essential to our functioning.

Our intuition is part of our wholeness. It is one of the "gifts" we have been given to help us navigate this life; it adds serenity when we heed it. How many mothers and fathers "feel" that something is going on with their children before their brains get the concrete message? How many of us know there is something wrong with a business deal when on the surface everything looks fine?

Intuition is not something that only a chosen few have been given. Intuition is buried deep inside all of us. Like many of our birth-given gifts, it gets better with practice.

Practice using your intuition. It helps to take some quiet time each day to let your inner being know that you're open to hearing from it. Pay attention to small feelings or stirrings inside your body. When an image or thought flies through your mind, write it down in your "intuition training booklet" (a notepad you've bought to carry with you). Don't feel pressured to "do" anything with your intuitions until you are ready. That will come later.

CELEBRATING COMPLEXITY

The intellect has little to do on the road to discovery. There comes a leap in consciousness all of it intuitive or what you will, and the solution comes to you and you don't know how or why.

ALBERT EINSTEIN

We human beings are such a marvelous mixture of processes, energies, and forces that to try to reduce us to simplistic ideas and processes is idiocy indeed.

We are not machines. We will *never* be machines. Regardless of how sophisticated science becomes, it will never be able to emulate the complexity of a simple human being.

Today is a good day to celebrate our complexity and our unreasonableness! There are times when we are not understandable to ourselves or anybody else. So be it. Isn't it great? We are not understandable! We are too complex to be completely understood. We are a conundrum. We are a paradox. We are a mystery. We are unfathomable. We are great!

This day, take a giant step toward enjoying your complexity.

MARRIAGE

Almost no one is foolish enough to imagine that he automatically deserves great success in any field of activity; yet almost everyone believes that he automatically deserves success in marriage.

SYDNEY J. HARRIS

What a true statement! I once heard someone say that assumptions are premeditated resentments. I wonder if this applies to marriage.

If we come into marriage with the belief that success is our marriage-right, we are setting ourselves up to be passive, resentful victims. With this assumption, we have, with great alacrity, removed ourselves from participation, leaving the outcome of the relationship to forces unseen and unnamed. No wonder so many marriages fail and so many people get angry about marriage. No one ever likes to be deprived of a "right."

We would do better to view marriage as a form of ongoing participation in life with someone we like. This view of participating with a loved one—with no attachment to the outcome—tends to result in a favorable outcome.

Write down your assumptions about marriage. It's good to look at them, perhaps even with your spouse. You may want to question some or all of them.

CHILDREN

A business society . . . always has in its children a large group of individuals who cannot make money and who do not understand (or want to understand) the profit motive. In short, they are subversives.

MARGARET HALSEY

How can we learn to live in balance when we see our children as subversives? Like all of us, children are sacred beings. Yet, if we do not recognize our own sacredness, it is quite unlikely that we will recognize the sacredness of our children. Children are not a means to an end. They are the embodiment of sacredness placed in our hands for safekeeping for a while. When we try to make children fit into the demands of our business society or see them as getting in the way of what needs to be done, we are in danger of perceiving them as subversives interfering with what's vital and important.

Even though we may need subversives in our lives to keep reminding us of what is important, when someone or something is seen as a subversive because of differences, we have lost touch with the need for differences to balance our lives.

Children are different from adults. Thank goodness! They can remind us to value differences and learn from them. They offer us a very personal opportunity to face our fear of differences.

Check out your attitude toward children . . . honestly.

TURNING THE SITUATION AROUND

When my workplace wanted to move me to another office sixty miles from my home, I didn't go into "victim." I looked for the solution.

UTTA

When we work outside the home, we have to deal with issues that come up in the workplace. Often there are questions of "displacement" of one kind or another. The job we have done for years has been given to someone else. Our organization wants to move us to a new, less convenient place. The building needs to be remodeled and we are going to be given a workspace in that seems impossible for us.

All of these instances give us the opportunity to move into being a victim or to start fighting and become a perpetrator. Neither solution looks too promising. What is the third option? Often, it is to stop, take a very long, very deep breath, spend some time with ourselves (not obsessing, just waiting with clarity), and then move into action.

While Utta was getting clear, she sent out some résumés to potential employers (having given some thought to what she *really* wanted to do), had some interviews, and landed a job that, for her, was much better than her previous job. She later realized that she had been dissatisfied with her old job for some time!

God does for us what we cannot do for ourselves.

Don't grumble; take action!

OUR HERITAGE

I had a heritage, rich and nearer than the tongue which gave it voice. My mind resounded with the words and my blood raced to the rhythms.

MAYA ANGELOU

In our busy lives, as we race through everything that needs to be done *now*, we rarely take the time to sit down and recognize and explore our rich heritage. None of us is without a heritage. We may not be familiar with it, we may have even tried to escape it, and, it is there.

Our heritage is an important part of who we are. It is the roots from which we spring and the lineage that helps give us definition. Our heritage is not only important to us: it is important to our children, and it is something we can share, explicitly or implicitly, with all with whom we come in contact.

In this time of homogenization and globalization, many of us have spent a lot of time trying *not* to be who we are. We have sought some "idealized image" and been willing to give up our heritage in order to be accepted by others and ourselves. Yet our heritage is still there, beckoning us to return to our wholeness.

Start exploring your heritage.

THE MESSAGE AND THE MESSENGER

Do not seek to follow in the footsteps of the men of old; Seek what they sought.

BASHO

It's good to have mentors. It is even good to have heroes and people we admire. Yet all too often we tend to confuse the message with the messenger. When we hear something we like from someone, when a message stirs something deep inside of us, we unconsciously conclude that if we emulate the messenger, we will somehow be privy to the riches of the information conveyed. Wrong! And, unfortunately, those who have stumbled upon vast pools of wisdom sometimes confuse themselves with the wisdom they have discovered.

Ultimately, the messenger is not that important. Behind that person are deep reservoirs of information and wisdom that are available to all of us, if we but take the time to seek them. The messenger is simply the person who opens the door or points the way. We are the ones who must walk the path for ourselves and plunge into the wisdom pools that are there for all of us.

Those who share their wisdom with us have had to seek for themselves. When we "seek what they sought"—rather than seeking them—we have embarked upon life's journey.

We need to learn to see the balance behind the messengers, thank them for their wisdom, and use it for our own journey.

Today, take time to see instances where you have confused the message with the messenger.

OUR LIMITLESSNESS
AND OUR LIMITS

Chaos is not the opposite of order: it is the potential from which order may arise; it harbors an order or orders not yet discerned, and it is the limit which order cannot violate and still be order.

ROBERT H. KIRVEN

I love this—"It harbors an order or orders not yet discerned, and it is the limit which order cannot violate and still be order." Isn't it exciting to find a grouping of words we can chew on for some time and still be challenged to new depths of their meaning? We need such challenges. We need to find phrases, ideas, concepts, and experiences that stretch us, push us beyond our ease, and plunge us into chaos so that we emerge again.

What an idea—order or orders *not yet discerned.* They are discernible. They are there. They exist. We just have not yet reached a place where we can see them. We have the potential. We have the opportunity to move into and understand another level of the unknown that is just waiting there for us. Isn't this exciting?!

And, chaos is the limit that order cannot violate and still be order. The unknown has limits it cannot violate, just as we have limits we cannot violate. Chaos has limits that move much beyond the limits of our minds.

Aren't you glad that we don't know everything yet?

Let your mind wander beyond its self-imposed limits. Experience chaos and come back enriched.

REALITY CHECKS

I was more and more confused and needed to confirm some sort of reality for myself. It was important for this woman to verify that I had been there.

OLGA KHARITIDI

There are times when we just need to make contact with something or someone outside of ourselves to ground us.

The airplane tips and we grab the armrests and put our feet solidly on the floor. We have just been a part of a crazy interchange and we need to ask someone who was also there, "Am *I* crazy or was *that* crazy?" We read the newspapers and we find comfort when a friend or spouse mutters, "The world's gone nuts."

There are times when we just can't do it ourselves. Whatever "it" is, ultimately we have to do it "for" ourselves and we don't always have to do it alone.

Even if it is just consensual reality, we find comfort in a shared reality when the ground beneath us is in upheaval. And let's face it, we all have times when the ground beneath us is in upheaval, whether it is the ground of our relationships, the ground of our work, or the ground of our being.

We need reality checks.

Who are your reality checks? We all need to find people we can trust to be our reality checks and a spirituality we can trust to be our reality check.

EXPEDIENCY

The immediate is often the enemy of the ultimate.

INDIRA GANDHI

We suffer from the disease of expediency. The quest to find the shortcut, the fastest way, the most convenient approach has become an obsession, especially for busy people. We are in constant search of the gimmick or trick that will give us an advantage. To do so is deemed smart and savvy. We content ourselves with the stopgap measure and manage with the makeshift. We pride ourselves on getting the job done and lose sight of how we have done the job.

There are two questions we need to ask ourselves when we settle for the expedient: (1) Do we feel good about ourselves and what we have accomplished when we have operated this way? (2) Have we lost sight of the ultimate? If our answer is no for the first and yes for the second, we need to take stock.

Ultimately, getting the job done may definitely not be more important than how we do it. We feel good when a job is finished. We feel great when we have done it in a way that was pleasant, growth-producing, and fun for everyone involved.

And more important, in the process of getting the job finished, did we keep sight of what is significant and ultimate? If we look down the line a hundred years, what's *really* important?

Never let expediency be the enemy of the ultimate.

Take a look at how you approach tasks. Try to keep the ultimate in mind.

SATISFACTION

Nobody's ever satisfied until they've been dead a good week.
LUCILLE KALLEN

What happened to satisfaction? We are all afraid to feel satisfied because we are deathly concerned that if we *are* satisfied, it will mean that we aren't moving on, aren't wanting more, better, faster, and harder.

Satisfaction is a breather given us for things going well. Say we finished a project. We need to let ourselves be satisfied. We have beautiful children. Why push? Evolve and grow together. We have a nice home. Enjoy it.

What a beautiful day it is (regardless of the weather!) when we take the time to stop, look around us, and breathe a sigh of satisfaction.

Of course there is always more to learn. Of course there is always more to do. Of course we can always grow and deepen. This doesn't mean that we can't afford ourselves the opportunity to be satisfied right now. Life will give us additional opportunities if we are alert to them. We don't have to struggle, suffer, and be dissatisfied into them. They'll come.

Try letting yourself have moments of satisfaction during the day. You might even find that someday you'll end up with a whole day of satisfaction.

CHORES

I hate chores. I hate chores. I hate chores. I'd rather do something more interesting.

SCOTT

Wouldn't we all! Chores can be boring at times, especially when we approach them as chores. There is just something about the word *chore* that elicits negativity in us.

I have a friend whose father's goal was to make enough money that he wouldn't ever have to do anything for himself. One of the results of this was that my friend developed very few skills for practical living; he was raised to pay someone to do everything for him. To his credit, he has learned how to do chores; he has even discovered that chores ground him.

Chores help us situate ourselves in time and space. They give us the opportunity to learn what we can do and what we can't do. They give us the opportunity for a kind of movement meditation in which we can do something and clear our mind and relax at the same time. Chores offer us the opportunity consciously to do nothing while giving our mind a break. What more could we ask of activities that present themselves routinely?

When you start resenting chores, stop to remember what they do for you (and how many chores others do for you). That thinking will restore perspective.

BEING GOOD AND BAD

Some are thought good and some bad, and both are wronged.
CUBAN PROVERB

What a burden it is to be seen as bad. What a burden it is to be seen as good. Both views distort and compress a very complex, multifaceted human being into a one-dimensional line.

Some of us have difficulty accepting our badness. We want to be good. We *try* to be good. And, when we can't pull our goodness off, we may be tempted to resort to a "con"—but only sometimes, because this would throw us into the "bad" category. Rarely do we stop to let ourselves realize what a burden it is to be considered good. When we have bad thoughts, bad feelings, or even bad behavior, we want to repress them, to hide them, even from ourselves. This is a burden.

Some of us have difficulty accepting our goodness. We are never good enough, no matter what we do; we could have done better. We have unrealistic expectations of ourselves, and when we fail, we resort to "I told you so. I'm no good." Even when we are good, we are suspicious of our goodness. We can just never leave ourselves alone.

We wrong ourselves and others when we see them as being exclusively good or bad.

We are humans. Humans are good *and* bad. We live in paradox, and we *are* paradox. The best thing we do may also be the worst thing we do. All we can do is bumble along the best we can, asking forgiveness and learning from our mistakes.

Accepting ourselves means accepting *all* of us.

When you do something you don't like, accept it, do what you have to do to right it, and move on.

RESTORING BALANCE

We need to go back to being people who think in terms of the needs of others. Learn to be kind in the Maori way, be grateful for what you have instead of asking for too much. Notice when your neighbor feels pain, sorrow, sickness. . . . We have to try to rebalance things.

ELLEMAIN EMERY

"We have to rebalance things."

What if each of us sees ourselves as someone who personally has to rebalance things? What if we take it directly upon our own shoulders to do what needs to be done to start rebalancing not only ourselves but also our society, the nation, and the planet?

Cultural change is only a bunch of individuals starting to do something different at approximately the same time.

In our small corner of the world, we can start to notice our neighbors—at home, at work, at church, or on the throughway. We can approach each with compassion, even if we actually *do* nothing. We can see them as people like ourselves, people who do the best they can even when it isn't what we would like them to do. We can notice when they feel pain, sorrow, sickness.

We can bring back balance as we respond to those around us.

Try noticing your neighbors in all spheres with compassion.

YES, NO, NEITHER

The single most dangerous word to be spoken in business is "no." The second most dangerous word is "yes." It is possible to avoid saying either.

LOIS WYSE

Balance may start not with our yeses or nos but with our maybes. "I'll sit with that" may be the most important phrase you will learn in your life.

Right! We live in a fast-paced world. That's all right. Right! People expect us to be able to think while we're running and give a quick answer. Right! If we don't perform, someone else will take our place. That's okay. Right! We demand of ourselves that we produce, produce, produce. So what? Is the world going to collapse if we slow down? Is everything an emergency? We throw our worlds out of balance with speed.

Some things just need to be pondered. There are times when we don't have a quick answer (or when our quick answer may not be our best answer). More often maybe than we would like to admit, we just are not ready to give an answer.

We have the right to say nothing. We also have the right to take three deep breaths and say those frightening and unacceptable words, "I don't know." We can utter, "I'll have to ponder that and get back to you," and still live to tell the story.

Try the above responses. And remember—when in doubt, don't.

ENDINGS

The adventure is over. Everything gets over, and nothing is ever enough. Except the part you carry with you.

E. L. KONIGSBURG

Endings are one of the areas in which we lose our balance the most. As busy people, all too often we don't want to take the time necessary to deal with endings. We prefer to create a crisis, generate emotion, overflow with adrenaline, and storm out, believing that we have constructed an ending. All too often what we have created, though, is a *scene*, not an *ending*. The ending process retreats beneath our consciousness, where it swirls around, affecting us more than we care to admit.

We had best learn to deal with endings, because our lives are made up of beginnings, endings, and times in between. Relationships end. We may continue in a new relationship with that same person and in order to do that, we must deal with the ending of the old relationship.

Jobs end. In most cases, it's probably time for a job to end when it does. Down deep we may know that, and yet we fight change as if it were limiting and bad.

It is only in acknowledging, accepting, and working through the change process that we are ready to welcome the new (and the new aspects of the old).

How do you handle endings? Take a look at them from the perspective of being part of an ongoing process and see what you see.

SUPPORT

I always wanted to be somebody . . . If I've made it, it's half because I was game to take a wicked amount of punishment along the way and half because there were an awful lot of people who cared enough to help me.

ALTHEA GIBSON

In order for us to feel (and be) balanced, we need to have support. We humans are group creatures. None of us really makes it alone, even though we may like to think we do.

For us to have all the energy we need to do our work—whatever that work is—we need support, especially emotional support.

Emotional support works best when it is an infinity sign—with the support flowing in some reasonably equal way between and among people. If some are always the takers and some are always the givers of emotional support, it just doesn't work very well. The givers get depleted and resentful (unless they have ascended!) and the takers eventually feel angry and beholden.

One of the ways that we can contribute to balance in our own and in others' lives is by learning how to give and receive support.

What's your giving and receiving support quotient? Be honest now: Are you unbalanced in this important area?

ENTERING THE HOLY

All our acts have sacramental possibilities.

FREYA STARK

When we treat everything we do with an awareness that all is holy if we regard it as such, we have a very good possibility of operating from a place of balance.

We have come to accept the misguided idea that certain things, places, and people, are holy, and others are not. This then gives us permission to treat the majority of our world—people, places, things, and acts—as if they were not holy. Nothing could be further from the truth. Everything—*everything*—has the potential for being sacramental and holy. Holiness is a perception within us; it is not a state "out there" somewhere.

Holiness permeates the everything of the everyday if we let it. Say we are busy and our children or a colleague asks us for something. We have the potential, in our response, to commit a holy act. Or say we sit down and face off with a desk piled high with paperwork. Again we have the possibility of a sacramental act. When we approach a sink full of dirty dishes, we can treat washing them as a sacrament.

We have so many opportunities every day to enter into a sacramental act. We may not always respond in a spirit of holiness, and yet when we do, it is worth it.

Start seeing everything around you and every act you do as potentially holy. See what happens.

CONTROL

Life is so constructed that we never get caught up.

ANNE

One of the ways we introduce and perpetuate imbalance in our lives is by pitting ourselves against the natural order of things. Life is set up in such a way that there is always something to do. Even when we die, we will not be finished. There will always be some loose ends left over—things over which we have no control. And, therein lies the problem.

We do not control life!

These words may come as a shock to some of us. Yet, they pierce to the very heart of the matter. Ultimately, we are not in control. Some of the greatest stress we inflict upon ourselves and others comes from our attempts to control things that just are not within our ability to control. We make every attempt to break our lives down into "workable" segments that we can complete, thereby feeding our illusion of control. Despite our efforts, however, things routinely get out of hand, thwarting our fondly held illusions and resulting in stress and frustration. Life is constructed to elicit our participation, not our completion. Life is an ongoing process. Work is an ongoing process.

Don't waste time fighting the natural order. Find ways to participate with those around you and in your life. Try something—every time you are tempted to try to control, find a way to participate.

EXHAUSTION

I gave in to exhaustion. I had such a great time.

SUZANNE

When was the last time you gave in to exhaustion? When was the last time you had a good time giving in to exhaustion?

Exhaustion is not a personal attack on our being by our bodies and nerves. Exhaustion is a natural consequence of living at the pace that most of us live. When we see exhaustion as natural, we don't get so angry with it. When we see it as a loving warning given by our body and spirit, we can let go of our resistance and give in to feeling exhausted.

There are just times when our head is tired, our muscles are tired, our bones are tired, and our being and soul are tired. Don't get sick. Just be exhausted.

Laze, lounge, veg, sleep, indulge. Balance will slowly creep back into your life.

Take the occasional exhaustion day. You'll need fewer sick days if you do.

BLESSINGS

May the great mystery make sunrise in your heart.
SIOUX BLESSING

How lovely to be given a blessing!

Blessings come gently to our eyes and ears, tenderly caressing our being with love and compassion.

Blessings move through the cracks in our soul, healing them as they pass through.

Blessings give us images to fill the voids caused by the wear and tear of the world.

Blessings are a very easy and inexpensive way to pass around great treasures.

Blessings lighten us and fill us at the same time, while demanding nothing from us in return.

Blessings can be given anytime, anyplace, openly or silently. It really doesn't matter, as both the blesser and the blessed are enriched.

Try spreading around some blessings, and see what happens.

TRUE HOLINESS

. . . our faults cannot hurt God. Nor will our failures interfere with our own holiness . . . genuine holiness is precisely a matter of enduring our own imperfections patiently.

SISTER THÉRÈSE OF LISIEUX

Did you feel some relief when you read that "our faults cannot hurt God"? I did. I never realized that I was concerned about the power of my imperfections, and I guess I was. I am also intrigued by the idea that our failures do not interfere with our holiness. It suddenly seems so self-centered to magnify the power of our faults and failures as if they were the center of the universe.

How often we find ourselves focusing on the negative and forgetting the positive. Say we give a lecture. Two hundred and ninety-eight people love us and two people hate us, and what do we do? We focus on the two negative responses and forget about the rest.

We do a million things right at work and overlook one small item, and we despair or get furious with ourselves. How could we have gone wrong?

We have friends who not only want us to admit when we have done something wrong, they want us to suffer for it, feel terrible forever, and be punished severely, preferably by ourselves. How are we to escape indulging in our failures?

We can practice enduring our own imperfections patiently.

Practice accepting reality graciously when you foul up: learn to apologize, make amends, and move on. Indulging in suffering and self-punishment will only push you deeper into self-centeredness; it will never foster true holiness.

FOCUSING ON OURSELVES

A man who reforms himself has contributed his full share towards the reformation of his neighbor.

NORMAN DOUGLAS

It's important to notice the amount of time and energy we devote to trying to change other people. Sometimes we are in denial about this tendency and try to convince ourselves and others that we really just accept people as they are. We hide reality from ourselves and others.

At other times we are forthright in our efforts. We believe that somehow, some way, we have been blessed with greater knowledge and wisdom about others than they have about themselves, so we unabashedly plunge in to straighten out their lives. The certainty of our conviction is second only to the determination of our actions.

Aren't we dear? Where *do* we get these ideas?

The basic truth is that the only person I can change is myself; the only person you can change is you. And quite frankly, that should keep us busy for some time to come. It could even be interesting and fun in the process.

We might notice that as we begin to change, those around us seem different. Some of them might even start to change themselves.

When our focus is on the wrong place, we feel unbalanced. When we bring it back to ourselves, life gets easier.

See if you're focusing on others and trying to change them. You may be subtle, so look carefully. With great honesty, evaluate how successful you have been at those efforts. See if you are ready to put the focus back on yourself.

LOVING

The story of a love is not important—what is important is that one is capable of love. It is perhaps the only glimpse we are permitted of eternity.

HELEN HAYES

All too often we become distracted by whether we are loved or not, and thus being loved becomes our focus. It's great to be loved; words are inadequate to describe the exquisite feeling of that experience. Yet, absolutely nothing can even slightly compare with the marvelous feeling of being the one who loves. The lover of our completion is ourselves.

When we allow ourselves to love—whether it is the loving of a pet, a child, another person, a tree, or all of creation—we have stepped into the pool of transcendence that flows above and beyond ourselves into the all-that-is. When we allow ourselves to love, to be the lover, we are indeed given a "glimpse of eternity."

It's much more risky to our well-being not to allow ourselves to love.

Be aware of how you feel when you are loving. Remember, that feeling is yours. No one but you can allow it to be there or take it away.

SPIRITUAL PROCESS

... spirituality, as the ancients reminded over and over again, involves a continual falling down and getting back up again.
ERNEST KURTZ AND KATHERINE KETCHAM

When we accept that balance and spirituality are not static states, we have gone a long way toward being ready to experience them.

Some popular beliefs support the illusion that the acceptance of a particular ideology will result in a state of perpetual bliss. This has not been my experience nor my observation. We can achieve states of balance and deep spirituality and our humanness assures us that the process of life (and we ourselves) will throw more challenges our way.

Spirituality doesn't guarantee us ease or bliss. Spirituality offers us the tools to deal with whatever comes along and helps us move back to a state of balance and deep connectedness.

The great spiritual leaders have not spent their energy teaching us how to be statically perfect. They have taught us how to deal with life in the deep faith that we can always return to spiritual balance. This is a profound and ultimately useful gift.

When we know that we will fall down again and again and that we can be taught the tools to get up and move on to a higher level of spirituality, we have faith. Falling down is not a failure; it is a spiritual opportunity.

Check out what you have been demanding of yourself spiritually. See if you can be more accepting of your and others' spiritual process.

WINTER

There is a privacy about it which no other season gives you . . . In spring, summer and fall people sort of have an open season on each other; only in the winter, in the country, can you have longer quiet stretches when you can savor belonging to yourself.

RUTH STOUT

Our bodies and our souls *need* the seasons. In spite of our climate-controlled homes, offices, and shopping malls, we are affected by the seasons.

Winter is a very special time. We can settle in and pull into ourselves— and the weather around us supports this. Winter is a time when the whole family can belong to themselves and each other. Winter is a time when breaks for warm, spiced cider, hot chocolate, or popcorn seem like necessities. Nature invites us to pull "into," whether it is into ourselves or into each other. The schedule may seem the same, and yet there is an open invitation to allow "longer quiet stretches."

We feel so much better when we allow ourselves to respond to the invitation of winter.

Get some cider, popcorn, warm blankets, wood for the fireplace—whatever supports your pulling into and belonging to yourself—and respond to winter.

AWE

At the moment you are most in awe of all there is about life that you don't understand, you are closer to understanding it all than at any other time.

JANE WAGNER

What an absolutely precious state awe is! When we are in awe, we approach the grandeur of the knowledge of our place in the universe. In experiencing awe, we allow the brilliance and wisdom of the child and the innocent to return to our awareness.

Awe and self-centeredness are mutually exclusive. When we are filled with awe, we are at peace with the knowledge that we do not and cannot understand everything. A peacefulness permeates our being, descending upon us with this knowledge. Awe lets us glimpse the vastness of creation with the awareness that we are part of it. Awe is a knowing that transcends understanding (and in fact does not *require* understanding).

Stars, sunrises and sunsets, and nature in all its moods are good releasers of awe. If we have trouble feeling awe, children are sometimes willing to help us (if we can admit that we need their help).

When our bosoms are filled with awe, our minds can relax for a while.

When did you last experience awe? Arrange for awe possibilities in your life.

PRAYER

Our prayers are answered not when we are given what we ask but when we are challenged to be what we can be.

MORRIS ADLER

When I was young, I remember being disturbed over whether prayers are answered or not. Of course, at that time, an answered prayer meant getting what I wanted. Then a mentor said to me, "Perhaps the answer is no." Well, that pushed me off dead-center, and I began to look at prayer differently.

Later I realized that I had been raised to be codependent with God, believing it was my duty to pray because God *needed* my prayers. Then I quit praying for a while and moved on to "Thy will be done"—a prayer that amounted to simple resignation, since God's will clearly was going to happen whether I "ordered" it or not. For a while I just was able to say, "Hello there," and that seemed okay. Then I began to have "buddy talks" with God. Finally, I realized what I had known as a child: that my life and my participation in it were the most profound prayer I could give.

In living life, I am always being challenged to be what I can be. I have come to see that spirituality is nothing more than participating fully; when I am participating in my life, I am living my spirituality and living prayer.

What made prayer so hard? . . . I did.

Look at the way you perceive prayer and the phases you have gone through with it. Try to articulate what is comfortable for you now with respect to prayer.

UNUSED MINUTES

I would willingly stand at street corners, hat in hand, begging passers-by to drop their unused minutes into it.

BERNARD BERENSON

If time is money, many of us have a growing wealth of unused minutes. It's not that we have to be *busy* to use up minutes; it's that we need to be *present.* Sitting and staring may be the most valuable use we make of our time. Unfortunately and paradoxically, our most unused minutes are sometimes those when we have been the "busiest."

Procrastination is a favorite time-waster of busy people. We spend so much time running around in circles avoiding the task at hand that we wear ourselves out. The myth about people who do too much is that they *do* too much. The *reality* is that busy people often do a great deal of procrastinating; they waste time and energy *avoiding* getting the job done while convincing themselves that they are working.

Rarely do we stop to realize how precious each moment is until some crisis befalls us. At those crisis times, we suddenly look around us and see that the world is painted in bright colors of beautiful hues. And we don't necessarily have to have a crisis to learn what is precious to us. When we truly focus on the precious, unused minutes become a thing of the past.

Stop today and see if each minute is alive for you. If not, return to being present to it.

GUIDANCE

There is a guidance for each of us, and by lowly listening we shall hear the right word . . . Place yourself in the middle of the stream of power and wisdom which flows into your life. Then, without effort, you are impelled to truth and to perfect contentment.

RALPH WALDO EMERSON

We have guidance! How peaceful we feel when we *know* that we have guidance. Though we have to make the choices, unseen forces accompany us, support us, and have more information than we do. We have to do this life ourselves, and yet we don't have to do it alone. When we remember this, a peacefulness floods our being.

What do we feel when we truly let ourselves know that we can put ourselves "in the middle of the stream of power and wisdom that flows into our lives"? Even if we struggle with the concept of God, are we willing to admit that there is something bigger than ourselves? Are we open to the possibility that that bigger wisdom is active in all creation? Do we have access to knowing more than we think we know?

We can let a celestial sigh escape our lips as we relax and ease into truth and perfect contentment.

We don't have to *know* it all. We don't have to *do* it all. We don't have to *manage* it all.

Take short breaks during the day and let the knowledge that you have help and guidance enter your consciousness. See what happens.

HAPPINESS

When one door of happiness closes, another opens, but often we look so long at the closed door that we do not see the one which has been opened for us.

HELEN KELLER

Happiness isn't the problem. It's what we do with happiness that keeps us out of balance.

First of all, we have a deeply ingrained belief that we deserve to be happy. That belief entertains and cajoles our conscious mind. Unfortunately, many of us, just under that conscious belief, have a whole pool of swirling feelings and thoughts that deny our belief in happiness.

Down deep, we see nothing that we have done to *deserve* happiness. Our lack of faith all too often convinces us that no one or no thing guarantees us this birthright. We become convinced that we have to *make* happiness for ourselves, seek it wherever we can find it—and that when we have it for a moment, we need to hold on to it as hard as we can, because someone is sure to want to take it away from us. We hold on to it with such tight fists that we squeeze it to death.

We have misunderstood happiness. It is always there waiting for us, regardless of our circumstances. We have but to see and open the door. Happiness is a process, not a thing. It comes and it goes. When we embrace it with open arms, it kisses us with the sweet brush of its tender lips, lingers a while, and leaves. And, it will return—sooner than we think, if we do not keep staring at the old door.

Take a look at the way you deal with happiness. See if some modifications are in order.

SEEING BEAUTY

Love beauty; it is the shadow of God on the universe.
GABRIELLA MISTRAL

One must remember to see beauty and to love it.

Rushing around doing too much has an effect on our vision, resulting in a specific and limited blindness. This particular kind of blindness is so gradual and subtle in its manifestation that we rarely are able to see it coming; and once it has established itself, we have the illusion that our eyes are seeing normally. The specific blindness of which I am speaking is the blindness to beauty around us.

Seeing beauty requires the ability to slow down and to notice. Seeing beauty depends upon the ability to see with more than the eyes and feel with more than the heart. Seeing beauty is the process of opening up our senses and our being not only to what is but also to what can be.

When we are too busy or too rushed to see beauty, we miss the signals that God gives us to look deeper and more lovingly into every image that comes to us. The puddles of water on the highway, the clouds crossing the moon, the wrinkles in the face of an old neighbor—all show us beauty.

Seeing beauty a beginning of balancing.

Are you becoming blind to beauty? It is everywhere, in everything and everyone. Stop, look around, and see if you can still see it.

ATTITUDES TOWARD CHILDREN

Indians still consider the whites a brutal people who treat their children like enemies—playthings, too, coddling them like pampered pets or fragile toys, but underneath always like enemies, enemies that must be restrained, bribed, spied upon, and punished. They believe that children so treated will grow up as dependent and immature as pets and toys, and as angry and dangerous as enemies within the family circle, to be appeased and fought.

MARI SANDOZ

What a powerful statement! Are we ready to take an honest look at the way we think about and relate to our children as one of the ways we create unbalance in our lives? Even if we disagree with the above statement, seeing ourselves through the eyes of another culture opens our minds.

Do we treat children like "pampered pets or fragile toys"? When they were born, did we look upon them as something we had accomplished and bask in the glory of it all? Was their birth a time of great humility and awe for the gift of love and responsibility we had been given? Do we see them as doing things (natural childhood things) to "get us"? Do we see their constant string of colds, sniffles, and flus as a personal attack on us and on the lifestyle we hope to maintain, with or without them? Is the imbalance they have introduced into our previously ordered lives due to who they are or to our reaction to them? These are good questions to ask ourselves.

Stop to take a look at your attitude toward children—yours or others'—and see if some changes are in order within yourself.

THE FOUR ELEMENTS

The fireside is the tulip bed of a winter day.

PERSIAN PROVERB

Earth, air, fire, and water are elements that the ancients recognized as basic and important. All are healing.

There is absolutely nothing more comforting on a winter day than the tickling flames of a real fire. Something about a fire in winter warms more than the body. Something about the jumping of the flames and the sound of crackling returns us to roots that go very deep.

We need basic elements in our lives to keep us grounded. We need to touch the earth and know it is there. We need to breathe clean air, letting our bodies remember the feeling of clear, clean air rushing into them. We need to find a way to reconnect with a warming fire, whether it's a fireplace, bonfire, campfire, or fake fire in an electric heater. And we need to feel and glory in the fullness of water on our whole bodies.

Something about returning to these four elements grounds us like nothing else can.

In winter, it is important to do things that warm your soul and your body. What can you do? A hot bath, a fire, something warm to drink . . .

LOVE

Love is the simplest thing in the world. Yet, we often make it the most complicated.

ANNE

Love is an energy flow between ourselves and our Creator, between ourselves and another person, between ourselves and our family, between ourselves and a group of people, between ourselves and our pets, between ourselves and nature—between ourselves and almost anything. Sometimes our pets teach us more about loving than anyone or anything in our life.

All too often we get crazy about love. When someone or something loves us, we get suspicious: "What do they *really* want?" We try to control it, and we want to make sure it never goes away. We want *all* of it, fearing that if the person who loves us loves someone else, maybe there won't be enough love for us. We want it to "fix" us. Instead of doing our own work with our own issues, we want love to make everything all right; secretly, we want our lover to give us what we never got from our parents.

We get so busy that we forget that love is a gift and that we are not in charge no matter what we do. We can try so hard to control love that we actually push it away. We can't *make* someone love us no matter how cunning and powerful we are. That's the truth of it.

Today, when you are given the gift of love—whether from a dog or a spouse— accept it, with gratitude.

LOSING OUR SPIRITUALITY

When I am being workaholic and rushing around, I find that I lose all contact with my spirituality, my Higher Power.

PETRA

Workaholism and other obsessive behaviors put us out of touch with the reality that we are spiritual beings first and human beings second. When we are busy rushing around, we shift to automatic pilot, becoming more and more divorced from our feelings, progressively losing touch with ourselves. And when we lose touch with ourselves, we lose touch with that spiritual center within us that links us up with the all-that-is, the Creator of the universe, the Power greater than ourselves that is inside of us all.

Our rushing and our busyness create a fog layer that encloses us, surrounding us with thicker and thicker layers externally and building denser and denser fog layers within. Pretty soon, we have lost touch with that which guides our lives.

We need contact with our spirituality to be the people we would like to be.

Whenever you find yourself rushing around, stop to get reconnected with your spiritual being. You'll notice the difference.

TRUTH

If now isn't a good time for the truth I don't see when we'll get to it.
NIKKI GIOVANNI

Truth is the great balancer. We have to deal with many levels of truth every day. These different levels involve the personal, the interpersonal, the familial, the workplace, the local, the national, the planetary, and the universal. All are interrelated and necessary levels. As in many other areas of growth and functioning, the place to start is with ourselves. All too often we put off exploring our own personal truth, telling ourselves that we have more important work to do, that the children are too young now and need our attention, that truth is something one thinks about when one is older, that seeking personal truth won't make any difference in our busy lives—and so it goes.

As busy people, we know how easy it is to put off the important things and focus on the little tasks that keep us scurrying around. In fact, we often convince ourselves that busyness and rushing are, in themselves, the truth.

Overdoing and rushing may be the truth of our lives, and yet they are not our own personal truth. However, when we recognize that we have made busyness our truth, we have taken the first step toward exploring our personal truths.

Sit down and list three things that are central to the truth of your life today and take a good, hard look at them. See if you would like to change them; and if so, how.

HOLIDAYS

I don't know how to "do" holidays. In my family, they were always a disaster.

HENRY

So many of us associate upset and even pain with the holidays that it is difficult to remember the idea of balance as we approach the holiday season. Many of us resort to our old friends—isolation and control—and just hope to get through it all. Frequently it is our families who trigger all our old, unresolved "stuff," and frankly, who needs it?

Having worked with the concept of balance for the past eleven months, we could approach the holidays a bit differently this year.

1.   *We can be open to approaching our family with love and compassion. We may not like the way certain family members behave, and yet we can remind ourselves that they are doing the best they can.*

2.   *We can "sandwich" what we anticipate might be particularly rough occasions between phone calls with people who would be supportive.*

3.   *We can arrange support groups of friends or visit twelve-step groups during the holidays.*

4.   *We can schedule alone times and times to give ourselves the spiritual and emotional support we need.*

5.   *We can be aware of our danger signals and respect them.*

6.   *We can pray.*

7.   *We can relax, have a good time, and let others deal with themselves.*

Happy holidays!

PRAYER

The ear of the great Master of Life, which is still open to my cry, will be penetrated with the invocation of blessing.

SHAWUSKUKHKUNG

Many of us, having had unfortunate experiences with organized religion, have thrown out the baby with the bathwater. For some of us who do too much, prayer is just one more thing added to a long list of too many things to do. Spiritual nurturing is often the first thing we drop when we get busy, estranging ourselves from our spiritual base right when we need it most.

Yet, somehow deep inside we know that whenever we make even the smallest attempt to reconnect, the other end of the connection is always open. Whenever we ask, we receive—though the answer doesn't always look like we thought it would look or how we wanted it to look.

Asking for blessing reconnects us with the Divine within us, which is an eternal fire always ready to be fanned, a spiritual spark warming and nurturing our being as nothing else can.

Skepticism is great. It keeps us on our toes and helps us learn, helps us get clear about what is right for us. The skeptic who is not open-minded enough to test out that questioning loses out.

Today, try a little tiny prayer: ask for blessing and give thanks for something. It can't hurt.

LOVING BEAUTY

Tell them how we loved all that was beautiful.
ANONYMOUS AMERICAN INDIAN

How important it is to love beauty! If we are open to seeing beauty, we find it all around us. When we look, we can see beauty in every face we meet. Every person, no matter how different he or she is from us, has a unique and special beauty.

How much the American Indians love the earth! There is so much beauty in every tiny piece of nature. The veins in the leaf of a tree, the bark of that tree, the rocks, even the patterns in the cracks of the sidewalk can have their own beauty if we are available to see them.

Just as beauty is in the eye of the beholder, ugliness is in the eye of the beholder. So much of what we see and experience reflects the attitude that we bring to it. Remember, attitude is contagious—positive or negative. We can contribute whatever attitude we wish to any situation.

Today, and each day, do some little act to make the world a more beautiful and better place. Pick up some trash, plant a seed, or bring flowers to the office. You'll be glad you did!

SILENCE

A heavy snowfall disappears into the sea. What silence?
FOLK ZEN SAYING

A heavy snowfall is something; it has existence. Yet as snow falls into the sea, it becomes nothing and participates in the silence.

The secret of balance is knowing *both* our somethingness *and* our nothingness. Each snowflake is unique and individual unto itself—a very special creation. Together, all these tiny special creations become a heavy snowfall capable of great beauty and of great destruction.

Yet as snowflakes are absorbed into the vastness of the sea, the individuality that was their uniqueness becomes an important part of a greater whole, resulting in a magnificent silence.

So it is with us! As we know and value our uniqueness, we also have the possibility of melding into and becoming part of the all-that-is.

Through our uniqueness we become part of the whole.

Today, seize the opportunity to practice the consciousness of the snowflake.

PEACE AND BALANCE

To know balance is to love peace.
ANNE WILSON SCHAEF

Balance is peaceful. There is no striving, no twirling, no unsteadiness in balance. Balance is not dead or boring; it is peaceful.

We people who do too much generally have drifted far away from peace. We have forgotten what peace feels like and therefore do not find ourselves contributing much peacefulness to our surroundings.

We all have the potential to know balance. Simply to *desire* balance is to begin to know. We can start with stopping, taking a few deep breaths, and letting the nervous energy drain out of us. We can let our minds become quiet, and we can make a commitment to ourselves to seek the peacefulness of balance wherever we are. We can open our hearts and minds to peacefulness. We can let peacefulness enter through the bottoms of our feet and flow up through our bodies with our breath and aliveness. We can breathe in peacefulness and breathe out agitation.

We can bring ourselves to a place where rushing, excessive adrenaline, and a frantic pace no longer feel normal or desirable.

To know balance is to know peace.

Try the above and see how you feel. There's no prescription and no right way. Find your way to bring peace within you. It may be walking in the woods or staring at a fire. The important thing is to find your own way.

ANGELS

I was talking to angels long before they got fashionable . . . So maybe you don't believe in angels, that's all right, they don't care. They're not like Tinkerbell, you know, they don't depend on your faith to exist. A lot of people didn't believe the earth was round either, but that didn't make it any flatter.

NANCY PICKARD

For much of the world this is a day of miracles. For all of the world this day and any day can be a day of miracles. Among the miracles in our lives are angels.

"Good heavens!" you say. "Why on earth is she writing about angels in a book on balance for people who do too much?" In order to live in balance, we need to recognize and live with both the seen and the unseen. In fact, as we do that, the unseen tends to become more visible.

Many years ago I didn't give much thought or credence to angels or spirit guides in my life. Then I happened to meet a world-renowned psychic, who quickly informed me that I had a ton of beings around me who wanted to help me but couldn't because I thought I had to do everything myself. (He was right about *that*.) He encouraged me to ask for something I wanted. "Parking places" came as the quick answer. "Parking places?" he asked. "Yes," I said, thinking that this would be a good scientific test. In the several years since then, I've had no trouble finding parking places. It's now a little joke between me and my spirit guides (angels). As someone who considered herself a scientist, I found it difficult to accept angels. Now it's not so hard

There are forces, beings, energies here to help us. Try learning to ask for help.

EXCUSES

We are responsible for our lives. When we accept that responsibility, our lives smooth out and get easier.

FORREST

How we resist taking responsibility for our lives!

- *I came from a dysfunctional family.*
- *I am an addict, what do you expect?*
- *I'm Scandinavian[Irish, Dutch, Swahili, whatever], that's why I'm this way.*
- *I was hurt way back when in a relationship, and I'm afraid to open up.*

Okay. All right. All this is true! And now what? Are we going to spend the rest of our lives hiding behind the excuses that culture has so graciously given us? If we do, we will not know balance.

There comes a point when we have to take responsibility for our own lives. All "those things" may be true, and yet we are right here, right now, and we have some choices. We can choose how we want to respond. We can acknowledge our feelings, honor them, work through them, and go on. We have so many possibilities, and the choice is entirely ours.

Take a look at areas in your life where you use excuses, thereby avoiding the balance you might have. See if you are ready to move on.

LITTLE THINGS

Let little things go.

ANONYMOUS

This could be the year that you decide to let little things go. If so, you will no doubt begin to find that not much is big stuff.

Does it really matter that the dinner is overcooked? Only if your ego is involved.

Does it really matter if you're late? Not if your peace of mind (and that of your family) is important. Does it really matter that you look just perfect? Only if you're willing to sacrifice happiness for effect.

This is a good time to let little things go, accept life on life's terms, and be open to what is. If we learn to respond to life with all the grace that is in us, grace will reward us back.

We can accept the timing and the process of everything around us. I always think of my toothpaste-tube experience. It was clear to me that I would be running out of toothpaste soon, so I bought a new tube, assuming I would need it right away. The medicine cabinet was small and *two* toothpaste tubes seemed a lot, so I focused my attention on using up the old one. That old tube just wouldn't run out of toothpaste. I started using more each time—no luck (and wasteful). Each time I used it, I thought surely the next time would be the last—for weeks, it seemed. I began to realize that something significant was going on between me and the tube of toothpaste. I wasn't thanking it each day for its generosity. I wasn't glad it was lasting so long. I wasn't thrilled when there was still more toothpaste. I wanted to hurry up and finish so that I could get on to the next tube.

Busy people do the same with their work and their lives.

Check out the toothpaste tubes in your life and try gratitude instead.

CHEERFULNESS

A happy woman is one who has no cares at all; a cheerful woman is one who has cares but doesn't let them get her down.

BEVERLY SILLS

What a marvelous distinction! We can be balanced without necessarily being happy all the time. We can be balanced without everything going perfectly all the time. In fact, maybe true balance has more to do with keeping our equilibrium *no matter what* than it does with trying to get all our ducks in order. Have we been paying so much attention to the ducks that we have forgotten to notice who was feeding them?

Can we be happy all the time? I sincerely doubt it. Can we deal in a balanced way with whatever life hurls at us, or return to balance rather quickly? Probably.

Approaching whatever is in front of us as cheerfully as possible certainly goes a long way toward keeping the doors to balance open (and toward making a return to balance).

Cheerfulness challenges our control, smokes out our negativity, and helps us rebound from the doldrums. Cheerfulness is pretty good stuff!

When the going gets rough, try some cheerfulness.

PEACE

The peace of men will settle the earth.

MARY SUMMER RAIN

There is no way we can heal the earth without healing the people. There is no way we can heal the people without healing the earth.

In Samoan medicine, when a person gets sick, the healer always looks at what is going on in the family, the village, and the culture. There is no concept of the person existing in isolation or out of context.

In Western culture, we give lip service to our awareness of the effects of toxic waste or of carcinogens in the food and air, and yet we really don't relate these problems to individuals. Nor do we systematically relate individual illnesses and imbalances to what is going on in the culture.

The culture and the individual are inseparable. They interact intricately, affecting one another. All too often we try to keep ourselves so busy that we can't really see what is going on.

Not all of us can change the world unless it *is* all of us, and, we can change our immediate environment. Let's take our work environment. What can we do to make it more conducive to a peaceful environment? Could we arrange the furniture differently? Could we add something, remove something? Could we bring in a footbath to use occasionally? Would certain scents help?

All of us can do things to make our living and working environments more peaceful. That peace will then seep into us.

ORDER AND CHAOS

You will thus find that chaos/order are not necessarily a pair of opposites, but that chaos provides a favorable condition to create new order.

DAVID B. ELLER

Did you ever notice than when you clean your house, things always get worse before they get better? We pull everything out of the closets and drawers, sort and pitch, organize, and then put things back together.

Or say we're starting a new project at work. We gather data and information (if we're a person who does too much, probably much more than we need!). It stands around in stacks, on pages of newsprint, with little notes pinned or taped to the wall, every conceivable surface covered. We feel completely overwhelmed. Then, suddenly, for no obvious reason, an order starts emerging before our very eyes.

If our houses and our offices seem to follow this simple wisdom about chaos and order, why not our lives?

The problem may not lie in order or chaos. The problem may lie in what we do with both.

The next time you are faced with chaos, remember the inherent order that lies within.

OUR HOLY INFINITE CENTER

Life is meant to be lived from a Center . . . There is a divine Abyss within us all, a holy Infinite Center, a Heart, a Life who speaks in us and through us to the world. We have all heard this holy Whisper at times. At times we have followed the Whisper, an amazing equilibrium of life, amazing effectiveness of living set in. But too many of us have heeded the Voice only at times. . . . We have not counted this Holy Thing within us to be the most precious thing in the world.

THOMAS R. KELLY

We can live in balance only when we are committed to listening to the whisper of this "Holy Thing" within us.

See if you feel a tingle of excitement when you read the above quote. I do. See if, in your reading of it, it touches some knowing deep inside of you—a knowing that lingers in the hidden recesses of your being and has whispered to you since you were a young child. See if all the busyness, excitement, and rushing around have muted this whisper. Remember times when you have ceased to listen—probably when the whisper disagreed with your self-will—and think about what resulted.

What is the most precious thing in the world to you? Let it guide you.

ACKNOWLEDGMENTS

I am one of these writers who always thoroughly reads the acknowledgments in every book. How can we ever acknowledge the people, animals, plants, and processes that have gone into the birth of a book? Once we start, the circles of support and love just keep expanding in our minds. Acknowledgments are so much like the deep acceptance of life. Everyone and everything—every success and every failure, every height achieved and every depth into which I have plunged—has contributed to this book.

Gratitude to the Creator—the spirit of life within all things and the God of all creation that makes everything possible—seems appropriate for first acknowledgment. I am grateful for all that has been given me, all that surrounds me, and all that comes through me.

I want to acknowledge Pete Sidley, who suggests, types, edits, and helps keep the joy of writing joyful. He's not only competent, brilliant, dependable, and efficient; he's great to be around.

I want to thank the rest of my family—Chuck, my husband, who appears with lunch when I lose track of time, and Roddy, my son, who always has said, "Go for it, Mom." My Aunt Jan, my mother's sister, continues to offer support as the only one left of that generation. Bobbi and Kerri have covered the office while I do my projects and both have fed me quotes and materials for pondering the meaning of balance. Bobbi, being an avid reader, has come up with fabulous references that I might not otherwise have seen. Even the cats and dogs in their infinite wisdom have contributed to this book.

I love being back with HarperSanFrancisco and am excited about working with Liz Perle, an association that has been on my wish list for many years. David Hennessy at HarperSanFrancisco has helped heaps. I also want to acknowledge my longtime agent, Jonathon Lazear, and his staff, especially Christi Cardenas, for their ongoing support.

And last but not least the international *Living in Process* network, which supports, loves, feeds, and challenges me. They are always open to hear new material and give tough, loving feedback.

I acknowledge the processes of my life (even doing too much!) that have led me here.

NAME INDEX

INDEX OF THEMES